THE UNICORN DIET

MK LORBER

Three
Pom
Press

ISBN: 978-1-7359717-0-4

CONTENTS

AN ODE TO DIET LANDIA

There is no Insulin Fairy.
Don't spend your hard earned money,
On those "super berries."
I'm not selling AdvoCare-y.

If this book is Too Long/
Didn't Read,
I just want to plant the seed.
Moving more and eating less is all you need.

It's not quite that simple, folks.
There is no spell, nor a hoax.
Stick around,
For my dad jokes.

It's science's turn,
To take a stand.
Let's leave Yo-Yo Diet Land.
And learn about beaver's anal glands.

YOU'VE BEEN WARNED—AN INTRODUCTION

Here are some fightin' words.

All diets work because they eliminate something.

Maybe it's a particular food. Perhaps it's an entire category of cuisine. Or they place restrictions on when you can eat. Do you like to eat mid-day? Too bad. Your feeding window is now between 2:00 AM and 2:16 AM.

Don't believe me? Look at what's out there.

Anybody remember the Atkin's diet? Sure, it's fun in the beginning. Bacon and eggs for breakfast. Bam! Bacon-wrapped sausages for lunch. Holla! I get to eat a hamburger patty for dinner? Sweet, come to mama. It's all fun and games until you have a layer of grease splatters permanently coating your kitchen.

What about eating like a snake? It's a new fad where dieters fast for 24-48 hours, then eat an enormous meal of red meat. With this approach you will undoubtedly lose weight, but I hope you like creating chocolate soft serve out the other end for the first 3 months.

There is even the infamous cabbage diet. For anyone not in-the-know, it's self explanatory. You eat the cabbage and only the cabbage. As a result, you lose all the weight and alienate your coworkers.

Extremes are easy. Moderation is hard. And long-term deprivation is just crazy sauce.

How long are you really going to last dining on celery, cucumbers, and air? It's tough to stomach (pun intended), but all diets eventually fail.

I am here to tell you that there is a different way to look at food; there is a different way to look at your body.

Buckle up, buttercup. We are going to learn some science. And do the maths. Don't worry. There is not a test at the end. Unfortunately, you can't skip to the appendix and find the answers either.

Don't let that scare you away. I'm not trying to teach *The Common Core*. <shudders> But we need to learn about thermodynamics, which is just a swanky word for the study of energy. Ultimately, food is just fuel for the body.

Until it isn't. There is also an emotional component to food. We use it as a reward when we are happy. Or as a drug for negative emotions.

Food is also a significant part of our traditions. We break bread with friends and family. And if we can put down our little glowing devices, we get to know one another over grandma's special lasagna.

So how can we keep our food culture intact but also improve our health? Or shed a few pounds without hulking out on our loved ones in the process? Science has already given us the answer. The knowledge is more than 60 years old. So why isn't it everywhere?

The answer—the science of weight loss isn't *sexy*. Yep, I said it. You can't slap a colorful label on it to sell more goodies in the supermarket. It's too straightforward to blend in a shake and sell as a part of a pyramid scheme. And we won't see a Super Bowl commercial with half-naked bodies dancing to *energy expenditure*.

As you will learn, extra fat is just energy your body stores for the zombie apocalypse. Don't see any slow-walking, reanimated mouth breathers? Great. Your body doesn't *know* that. It's out here making sure you have enough energy to live yo' best life.

While we are at it, let's radically reframe your mindset. You are not fat. Maybe you have extra fat. But fat is not an adjective that defines you. It is not *who* you are.

$$\sim$$

Here's how I've laid out this book.

One, I put important things in bold, so you don't have to scrounge up a highlighter.

Two, there are infographics throughout because sometimes books for grownups really have too few pictures. And some of us learn better with a little visual aid and color in our life.

Three, you are going to meet my friends No-Drama Llama and Myth-Busting Mermaid. They are a much more reliable source of information than Jenny, your old high school pal selling sweat gel on her snapchatter, insta-story page.

Four, I'm going to make you put some skin in the game. I will give you homework and actionable items. I can hear you groaning already, but trust me. You will be better and wiser for completing these steps.

Five, I break down the science into easily understandable chunks. Don't fret. I've defined all those swanky terms so someone that slept though high school biology 20 years ago can still follow along.

Six, this is not a recipe book. I'm not going tell you what to eat. And I won't tell you what foods are off limits. There are no superfoods, nor evil villains. Except trans fats. They can go kick rocks.

Seven, this sure as heck isn't a juice cleanse, and this is not a front for selling vitamins or supplements. There is no need to spend $300 plus on that fancy kitchen appliance when you have a liver.

Eight, this is not a 6-week reboot, nor a 90-day challenge. There are plenty of those over-priced plans out in the diet universe. You didn't put on the extra weight in a month, so it's going to take longer than that to get rid of it.

Nine, we will learn about the components of our food, how the body stores and uses nutrients as energy, and how to calculate what you are eating and burning. I touch on metabolism myths, preventing that hangry feeling, and scheduling diet breaks. Toward the end, I dabble in some softer topics, covering stress, sleep, and goal setting.

Ten, there will be lists. My brain thinks in bullet points. Fortunately for our topic, it works nicely to compress broad subjects into manageable segments. Also, I needed a number ten to round out this list. Sorry, not sorry.

∾

Straight talk. Dr. Google failed me. I'm just another exhausted, middle-aged parent who had to figure this out on her own. I have just enough common sense to know there is no shake or superfood that is magically going to melt off the love handles. I suffered through just enough schooling to smell the dung pile of diet drivel on the inter-webs from a mile away. Finally, my daddy passed along just enough bravado to put what I've learned into this book and to launch it into the cesspool that is nutrition media.

So come at me, diet zealots. Bring your emotional arguments, your one-off anecdotes, and your close-minded dogma. I have science in my corner.

For everyone else, I hope you find something useful in my words.

Cheers, Dear Unicorns,
Melissa

PS and a Disclaimer:
Going through the editing process, one thing is clear. I talk about poo, a lot. It's unintentional but not unexpected, since I live with four young children. While I promise there are no fart jokes, I can't guar-antee that I didn't slip in a yo' mama somewhere.

PPS and another Disclaimer:
The science of weight loss is straightforward, but often rather dull. At the beginning of most chapters, I've included some interesting (and slightly inappropriate) food facts. While I've kept my proverbial toe on the right side of the politically correct line, it still may be slightly offensive to some readers. Apologies in advance to those who don't share my sense of humor. My intention was to lighten things up a bit. If you get nothing else out of this book, you will kill it at the next trivia night on food history questions.

PPPS and a more serious disclaimer:

This book is not for teenagers. You are still growing, changing, and figuring out life. Nor is it for pregnant or nursing mamas. You are incubating and raising small humans; thus, you have different fuel demands. Individuals with eating disorders or body dysmorphia need not read it either. Please start or continue your journey under the care of a trained physician. Folks with specific dietary needs because of a medical condition, listen to your doctor. Don't take dietary advice from someone like me who uses cartoon animals to illustrate her points.

1

MACRONUTRIENTS (WITH A TINY DOSE OF MICRONUTRIENTS)

There once was an ad campaign offering a free box of Kellogg's Corn Flakes to any woman who winked at her grocer.

Did you know that masturbation was once thought to cause 39 different maladies? Have teenage acne? Must spend too much solo time in the bedroom. Suffer from epilepsy? You need to get your hands out of your pants. Many moons ago, Dr. John Harvey Kellogg wrote a book prescribing a lifestyle of fresh air, a diet devoid of rich foods, and a strict adherence to sexual abstinence as the cure for patients who suffered from their lustful endeavors.[1]

Many of you might recognize the last name, Kellogg. Yes, this barrel of laughs brought us Corn Flakes, "a healthy, ready-to-eat anti-masturbatory morning meal."

The only thing that Corn Flakes compelled me to do as a young adult was to dump the entire mushy mess down the drain and sneak a pop tart. Dr. Kellogg was not the marketing guy in the family. It was his brother who popularized the cereal by adding a little sugar to the original recipe. I'm sure leaving off any mention of its original purpose also helped matters.

No-Drama Llama Rule:
Don't take nutrition advice from anyone who assigns morality to a particular diet.

~

Proteins (P), carbohydrates (C), and fat (F) are the principal components of our food—the macronutrients. The term "macro" denotes quantity, as these three are all measured in grams. Most of us don't eat these in pure forms; our food is a combination of P/C/F. One hundred grams of chicken is not one hundred grams of protein, despite what gym bros might try to sell you. Nutrients can be further classified as either essential or non-essential. The body does not make essential nutrients, and we are required to get them from our diet. Let's dive deeper into these three categories.

The Heavy Hitters

Protein
Every cell in the body requires protein for survival and function. Protein molecules play many roles. They serve as structural components in connective tissues such as bone, muscle, and cartilage.

Proteins act as enzymes in chemical reactions and as messengers in chemical signaling. Pepsin is a good example of an enzyme. It aids in the digestion of our food. Enzyme is just a swanky word for something that speeds up a process.

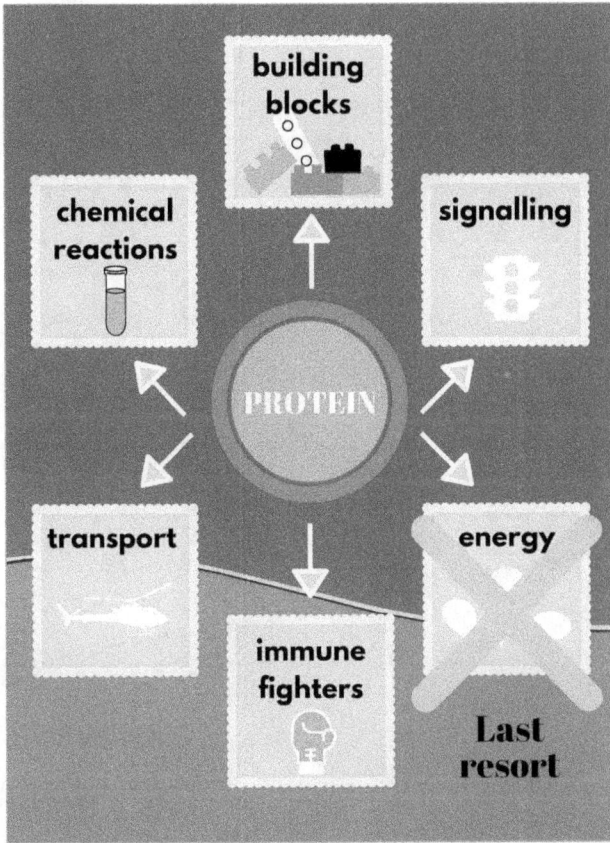

Antibodies are proteins that bind harmful pathogens and work with the immune system to expel them from the body. Imagine putting a virus in a headlock and taking it outside.

Finally, proteins can act as transports. Hemoglobin is one prominent example. Found on red blood cells, it transports oxygen from the lungs in the bloodstream.

Proteins are complex molecules assembled from strings of amino acids. Amino acid is just a swanky term for the building blocks of proteins. Our body needs 20 types of amino acids. However, it does not make 9 of them, so we must get them from our diet.

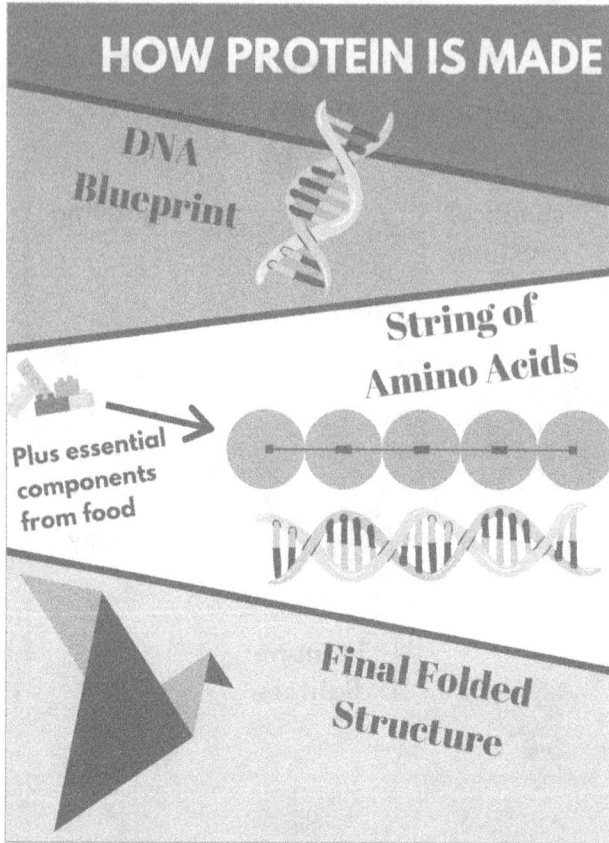

HOW PROTEIN IS MADE

DNA Blueprint

String of Amino Acids

Plus essential components from food

Final Folded Structure

Consuming protein is a requirement for all humans. Protein from food is digested in the stomach. Acid breaks down the larger structure into smaller sections (or chains of amino acids called peptides). Degradation continues in the small intestines, and the final bits and pieces pass through the intestinal wall to enter the bloodstream.

~

These small fragments circulate throughout the body for use by various tissues. Tissue is a swanky word for a group of similar cells that perform the same function.

Proteins are responsible for many critical tasks in the body, but we do not store them as fuel. The last thing the body wants to do is breakdown all the work it just put into manufacturing protein structures and burn them as energy. A builder doesn't want to remove interior walls of a house to burn as firewood, but he will use them if he needs the heat to survive.

**The body does not store protein for energy;
there is no protein silo.**

Because there is no storage location, it is important to consume protein daily. What is the minimum amount? That varies per person and depends on multiple factors. For instance, pregnant women have higher recommendations than adults of equal size.[2] Are your hobbies physical? You will need more protein than the average couch potato.[3] Have an illness or injury? The body needs extra energy to fight off infection and repair structures.[4]

Aim for 1 gram of protein/lb of body weight.[5, 6]

This number increases if you are lactating, pregnant, ill or injured, or taking part in strenuous activity.

Don't dip below 50g of protein a day.[7]

This is the bare minimum. I cannot stress this enough. It represents the threshold for survival and does not imply optimal health. Remember, we cannot manufacture 9 of the 20 amino acids in sufficient quantities.

Homework time: Find your favorite sources of protein and learn different ways of preparing them. For extra credit, research those 9 essential building blocks, discover which foods contain them, and make a list of your favorites.

Fats and Cholesterol

Who doesn't love a villain? Every hero needs an adversary. Think how boring stories, tall tales, and novels would be without this crucial character. News articles are no exception to this rule. In mainstream diet media, cholesterol is the proverbial scoundrel. Want cholesterol's side of the story?

The truth—cholesterol is essential for most cells and tissues. It provides structural integrity to cell membranes. The small, ringed molecule is a precursor for the synthesis of vitamin D. Synthesis is just a swanky word for making big stuff from smaller pieces. Cholesterol also serves as the base for steroid hormones such as cortisol, estrogen, and testosterone.

Our liver makes most of the cholesterol required. We consume the rest from our diet, mainly from meat and dairy products. This is a balanced system in healthy individuals. If dietary intake of cholesterol increases, then the liver decreases production. If one side of the scale goes up, then the other goes down.

After a meal, cholesterol gets absorbed through the small intestine and stored in the liver. It cannot travel freely in the bloodstream, so it hitches a ride around the body on carrier molecules, called lipoproteins. The body assembles these complexes in the liver. They are a combination of proteins, cholesterol, and triglycerides. Triglyceride is just a swanky word for a lipid (or fat) with 3 chains attached.

Have you ever read a copy of your blood tests? It looks like alphabet soup. My eyes cross from so many acronyms. Scientists love to classify things, and cholesterol is no different. Medicine divides lipoproteins into categories based on the amount of protein in the complex.

High-density lipoproteins (HDLs) transport cholesterol from cells back to the liver. They have the largest amount of protein. Doctor's assign them the label of "good" cholesterol.

Low-density lipoproteins (LDLs) haul cholesterol from the liver to the rest of the body. They have less protein than HDL. We know them as "bad" cholesterol.

Very-low density proteins (VLDLs) have a sizeable amount of triglycerides. They deliver these lipids to awaiting cells.

For some folks, high cholesterol increases their chance of having a heart attack or stroke. Hyperlipidemia is just a swanky medical term for high levels of cholesterol. It develops in two ways. You either inherit it (thanks, mom and dad), or it develops alongside other diseases, such as diabetes.

Diagnosed with hyperlipidemia? Follow the advice of your doctor. There are specific guidelines for the amount of cholesterol allowed in your diet. I shouldn't have to say this, but your physician is way smarter than an author who uses a mythical creature to help advertise her diet book.

∿

Let's take a look at fats and lipids. Lipid is just a swanky word for molecules that don't dissolve in water. Think of a lava lamp, with colorful lipid blobs floating in a water-filled container. In this book, I interchange the terms fat, lipid, and oil.

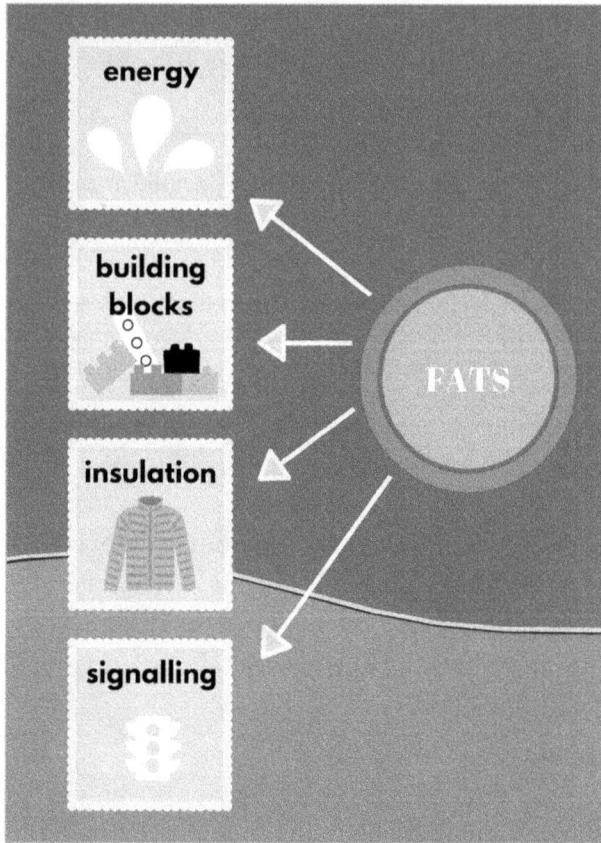

The body burns fat in our food for energy or stores it for later use. Reality weight loss programs prove that fat storage is virtually unlimited. We also use lipids as chemical messengers, as insulation, and as the building blocks of cell membranes. Lipids fall into one of three categories.

Triglycerides have a backbone, a ring-like structure called glycerol, plus 3 fatty acid chains. It reminds me of a wind chime with 3 chains hanging straight down. These molecules act as energy or energy storage. Triglycerides also provide insulation, your fat parka.

Phospholipids are fat molecules with a head plus 2 chains. They form most of the cell membrane. Think of old-fashioned wooden clothespins.

Finally, sterols are lipids with a ring-like structure and no chains. In case you slept through the last section, cholesterol falls into this category. Remember, it strengthens cell membranes and serves as a backbone for steroid hormones.

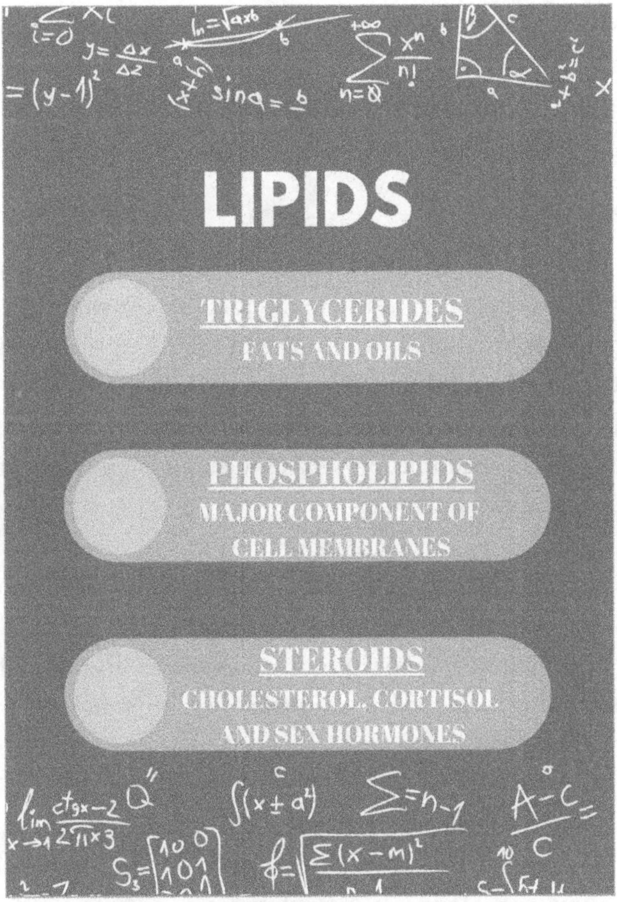

LIPIDS

TRIGLYCERIDES
FATS AND OILS

PHOSPHOLIPIDS
MAJOR COMPONENT OF
CELL MEMBRANES

STEROIDS
CHOLESTEROL, CORTISOL
AND SEX HORMONES

Fat from food is digested and absorbed in the small intestine. The liver produces bile that the body stores in the gallbladder. Bile emulsifies the gelatinous blob of fat that enters the small intestine from the stomach. Emulsify is just a swanky word for combining two things that don't normally mix. This creates smaller, more manageable lipid droplets.

Of note, fat-soluble vitamins A, D, E, and K require bile for absorption.

The smaller particle size allows the enzyme, lipase, to chop off the fatty acid chains from their glycerol backbone. Snip, snip, snip. The lymph system transports these smaller end products to the liver. After repackaging, the new lipoproteins move freely in the bloodstream, either for immediate use as energy or long-term storage in fat cells.

~

There are four types of fat found in the food we consume. Researchers classify them by the shape of their fatty acid chains and their state of matter at room temperature. While these categories are one way to group fat, keep in mind that food often contains more than one type. For example, pork has saturated fat, monounsaturated fat, and polyunsaturated fat.

Many of you have heard of trans fats in the news. Unlike cholesterol, they truly deserve all the bad press. Most trans fatty acids are man-made by bubbling hydrogen through oil to artificially straighten out their chains. This makes them semi-solid at room temperature. Hello, spreadable margarine.

Food manufacturers have added these oils to processed foods because they are inexpensive and increase shelf life. Fast-food restaurants use them to fry foods because they last longer than naturally occurring oils.

Unfortunately, consumption of trans fatty acids increases your risk of heart disease.[8] They also promote inflammation, add excess fat around organs, and may lead to insulin resistance.[9, 10]

There is no recommended daily dose for trans fat, so check the nutrition information of your favorite treats. Always look at the ingredients list for "partially hydrogenated oils," even if the amount on the label is zero. There is a sneaky little loophole where manufacturers can round down if the amount per serving is less than 0.5 grams.

Saturated fats are our next category. They are solid at room temperature. Think of the marbling in a piece of steak or the weird squishy stuff on chicken skin. Because saturated fatty acid chains are naturally straight, they have a higher melting temperature. These are the fats that make food taste amazeballs. Very lean athletes may benefit from saturated fats to improve hormone balance.[11] We find saturated fats in animal and dairy products along with coconut and palm kernel oil.

A word of caution: Saturated fats *may* raise blood cholesterol levels.[12] Folks with hyperlipemia should limit the amount consumed. See also: Your cardiologist is smarter than I, so listen to your doctor.

Our last group is unsaturated fatty acids. There are two distinct kinds, and the kinks in their chains make them liquid at room temperature. Monounsaturated fatty acids (MUFAs) have a single kink in their chains, whereas polyunsaturated fatty acids (PUFAs) have multiple kinks. They are both considered healthy fats.

We find MUFAs in plants, nuts, and eggs. They are also in avocados, olives, seeds and seed oils. Adding them to your diet may be beneficial in reducing blood cholesterol and triglyceride levels.[13]

Chances are you have heard of the two main PUFAs: Omega-3 and Omega-6. Both are essential, but the body requires more Omega-3 than Omega-6. For trivia night, the number refers to the location of a particular kink in their chain.

Ready for some more acronym word vomit? Strap in. The most common Omega-3s are ALA, EPA, and DHA.[14] The body converts ALA to EPA/DHA, but the process is not efficient and worsens with age. So slow your role on flax seed, unless you really enjoy the flavor. The best source for EPA and DHA are oily fish. We find ALA in nuts and seeds.

When you think of Omega-3s, I want you to think of brains. Brains, brains, and more brains. Not the gore of Halloween, but the complicated, healthy ones in an intact skull. Omega-3s are vital to brain development in infants and to preventing dementia later in life.[15,16] For all the stages in between, they reduce symptoms of mental illness, including depression and anxiety.[17]

Scientists also found a link between Omega-3s and a decrease in heart disease.[18] They are important for bone health and reducing inflammation from chronic disease.[19] Chronic is just a swanky medical term for something lasting a long time. Initial research shows Omega-3s likely preserve strength and enhance recovery from stressful situations.[20]

In clinic, I routinely prescribe higher doses of Omega-3s for my inflammatory dry eye patients. I usually start them on a high dose, between 3-4 grams daily, for 90 days. Once the condition is better controlled, the dose tapers to 2 grams, indefinitely.

For all the beating its reputation has taken, Omega-6 is still an essential nutrient. Your body requires it for optimal health, and we must get it from the food we eat. The most common Omega-6 is linoleic

acid (LA).cWe convert it into ARA, which breaks down into pro-
inflammatory mediators, or recruiters.[21]

Inflammation is a normal part of our immune system. If something
attacks the body, the body is going to punch back.cThis should be a
quick and finite, in medical jargon—an acute response.cOnce the
attacker is subdued and the tissue heals, the inflammation subsides.

However, if the mediators hang around too long, it can change the
style of fight.cAn acute response is like a controlled boxer executing a
meticulous game plan. Jab. Jab. Cross. Quick pivot to avoid their left.
If the fight goes on too long, the boxer may fatigue or return punches
wildly just to make it to the end of the round. This is chronic inflam-
mation.cThe body is simultaneously fighting an attacker but racking
up collateral damage by destroying some tissue around it.

Experts cannot agree on a ratio of Omega-3: Omega-6, but it's safe to
say the Standard American Diet (SAD) is too high in Omega-6.[22]

Homework time: Make a list of excellent sources of Omega-3 fatty
acids. Look at your current eating habits. Do you see a trend toward
Omega-6? Is there a simple way to reduce the amount? How can you
include more Omega-3s? Here are my recommendations for daily
targets:

For females, aim for over 1 gram of Omega-3s daily.

AND

**For males and pregnant/nursing females, aim for over 1.5 grams of
Omega-3s daily.**[23]

Demonizing Omega-6s is a prime example of bloggers, journalists,
and authors cherry-picking one type of food, nutrient, or eating habit
and using scientific information to make their *sensational* case.

Usually, it's selling a book or driving traffic to their website.cI don't hate the hustle; I just hate the game.cWith Omega-6s, it really can be "too much of a good thing." Here's the rub though, two things can be true at the same time. In our case,

Consumption of Omega-6 is essential.

AND

Most should reduce the amount of Omega-6 they are consuming.

Unfortunately, this is a very common tactic in social media nutrition universe. I implore you to use your bunk filter here and unfollow anyone who vilifies a class of nutrients that the body deems essential. Beware, con men create spin and are very good at cherry-picking data. The exception here is trans fats; they can go kick rocks.

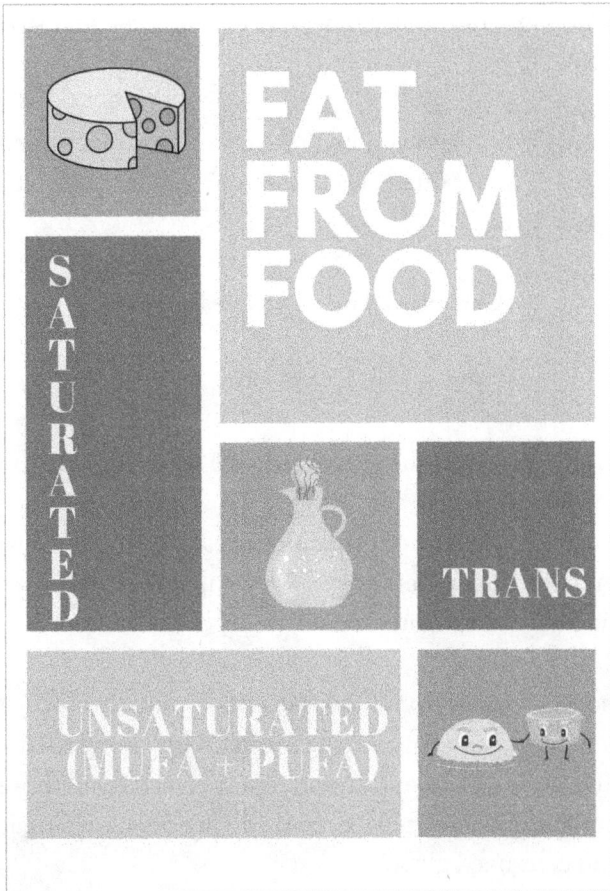

Carbohydrates

Le sigh. Can I just poke myself in the eyeball instead of discussing this? No? F-I-N-E. I can't think of a more polarizing topic in dietary wars than carbs. Low-carb this, high-carb that. Carb cycling. Good carbs, bad carbs, red carbs, and blue carbs.

Our ancestors didn't eat banana nut bread with a simple sugar glaze, so there is no way our body can handle the intense insulin spike. <eye roll> Get out of here, Paleo Patty, with your almond flour banana pancakes, drenched in maple syrup. I'm sure that's exactly what our ancestors ate. Congrats on bio-hacking, or whatever, that strand of ancient DNA.

There are only two things you need to remember from this section, and they are simultaneously true. The rest is just nomenclature and defining basic terms.

Carbohydrates are not essential.

AND

Carbohydrates are the preferred fuel source for the body.

Sure, you can survive without consuming carbohydrates. But do you really want to try? Be honest, here. How long do you think you will last cutting out your favorite treats?

In the absence of carbs from food, the body produces glucose through a process called gluconeogenesis. Why? Some tissues still require glucose as a source of energy. I'm speaking to all those keto and low carb enthusiasts here. Even if you are only burning fat for fuel, certain cells need glucose.

Here's something to consider. The body cannot make enough glucose to fuel high-intensity, explosive exercise. I'm talking about powerful movements. Sprinting and jumping. Swinging a bat or club. Tackling an opponent. So if you want to dunk in someone's face or beat your opponent to the ball, eat your carbs.[24]

PUBLIC SERVICE ANNOUNCEMENT

CARBS ARE NOT ESSENTIAL

BUT PERFORMANCE IS IMPROVED WITH INTAKE

PUBLIC SERVICE ANNOUNCEMENT

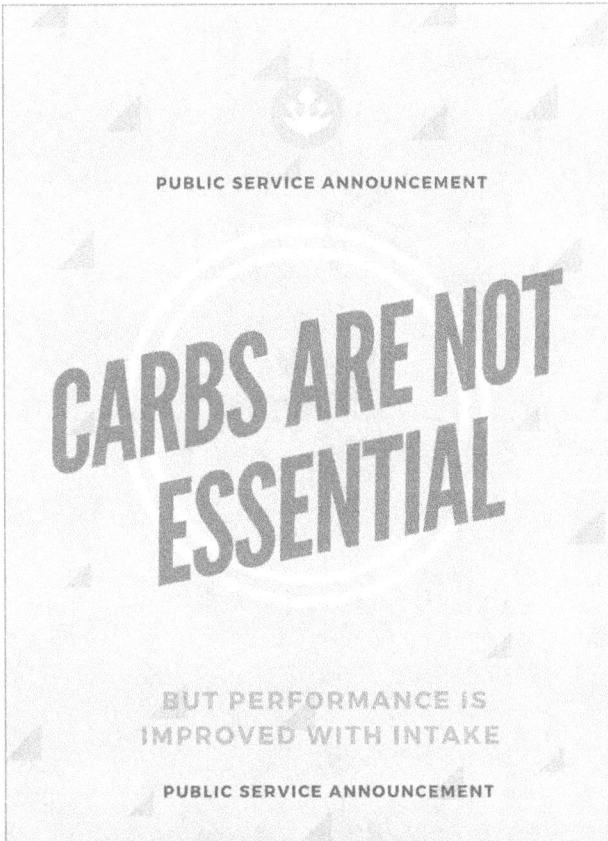

We classify carbohydrates by the number of saccharide units. Saccharide is just a swanky word for sugar.

Monosaccharides are single rings or units. This class includes glucose (blood sugar), fructose (fruit sugar), and galactose (milk sugar).

Disaccharides are double sugars or two linked rings. The most common examples are sucrose (table sugar), lactose (milk sugar from glucose plus galactose), and maltose (beer).

Long chains of sugar rings are polysaccharides. For our discussion, this includes starch in food and glycogen in the body.

SACCHARIDES

MONOSACCHARIDES
GLUCOSE, FRUCTOSE, AND
AND GALACTOSE

DISACCHARIDES
SUCROSE, LACTOSE,
AND MALTOSE

POLYSACCHARIDES
STARCH IN FOOD
GLYCOGEN IN BODY

Scientists also classify carbohydrates as either "simple" or "complex." They base this on how quickly the body digests them. We process sugars with fewer rings more quickly than those with longer chains. Because simple carbs need fewer alterations, they enter the bloodstream and raise blood glucose levels more rapidly than complex polysaccharides.

The body converts carbohydrates to glucose.

AND

The complexity of the chain determines the speed of entry into the bloodstream.

∾

Let's chase a white rabbit down its hole. Diabetes is an increasingly important public health issue. Nutrition circles throw around the terms Glycemic Index (GI) and Glycemic Load (GL) when discussing "good" carbs and "bad" carbs. These terms assist the diabetic patient with making informed food choices. But like any tool, they have their limitations.

Glycemic Index is a score determined by how a particular food will affect blood glucose levels immediately after consuming it. We compare the score to glucose (assigned a value of 100). For example, the index compares 50 grams of carbohydrates from watermelon to 50 grams of carbohydrates from glucose. The GI score of watermelon is high, coming in at 72. However, it takes over 5 cups of watermelon to reach 50 grams of carbs. Personally, I have no problem throwing back that much on a hot, summer day, but I realize that probably isn't a normal serving size for most.

Welcome, Glycemic Load. Scientists created GL to take into account the actual recommended serving sizes of food. For example, we compare 50 grams of carrots (not carbohydrates) to 50 grams of glucose. Now the scores make sense.

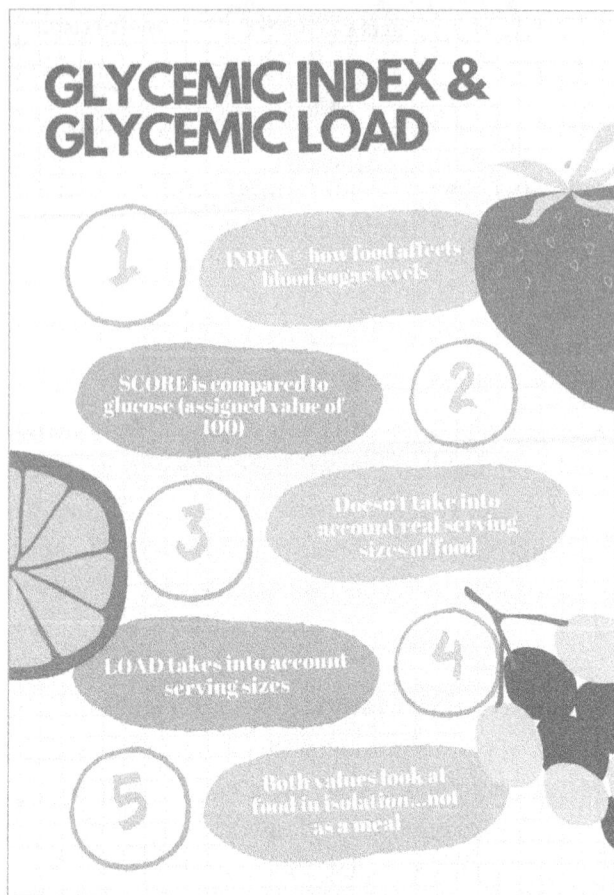

GLYCEMIC INDEX & GLYCEMIC LOAD

1 INDEX - how food affects blood sugar levels

SCORE is compared to glucose (assigned value of 100)

2

3 Doesn't take into account real serving sizes of food

LOAD takes into account serving sizes

4

5 Both values look at food in isolation...not as a meal

These scales serve as a starting place to learn about blood glucose control. I still remember the time when I discovered that pasta was "sugar." Education is key here. Most of us didn't study carbohydrates in school. Remember, GI and GL have limitations. Mainly, they only look at foods in isolation. They don't take into account the entire meal, which usually also contains proteins and fats.

∼

Do you ever feel tired after a carb-heavy meal? Have trouble sleeping on an empty stomach? My inner diva gets stabby sometimes if my blood sugar drops too low. There is a reason those "Hungry? Grab a Snickers" commercials resonate so well. Ever wonder why?

Cue serotonin—the "feel good" chemical. Serotonin plays many roles in the body. In our brains, it regulates mood, sleep, and appetite. There is a complex relationship between the carbs you eat and your serotonin levels.[25] Here is my oversimplified take on the events:

- Eats carbs. Nom, nom.

- Tryptophan enters the brain. You know, the one everybody talks about at Thanksgiving.

- Serotonin increases.

- All the dopey feels.

In science circles, there is speculation that very low-carb diets *may* decrease serotonin levels.[26] For patients with depression, this is problematic. As always, please be responsible and partner with your healthcare provider for advice on diet and mental health. For those not suffering from mental illness, my advice is to monitor your moods and note any changes that trace back to carb consumption. Nobody wants a stabby Susan.

The Flyweights

Fiber
Ah, fiber, the redheaded stepchild of the culinary world. Forgotten and often neglected, it's just plant roughage your body can't digest properly. Fiber is not essential, but it sure makes parts of life much easier.

The insoluble kind doesn't dissolve in the digestive tract and has a one-way fast pass straight through the other side. Its claim to fame is increasing stool bulk, an often-thankless job.

Soluble fiber dissolves in water. During digestion, it forms a blob, called chyme, which slows the emptying of the stomach. This promotes glycemic control and decreases blood cholesterol. To a tiny degree, chyme interferes with nutrient absorption because the digestive enzymes cannot travel through the muck and reach their target. On the flip side, foods high in fiber (think fruits, veggies, and grains) contain high amounts of micronutrients, vitamins, and minerals.

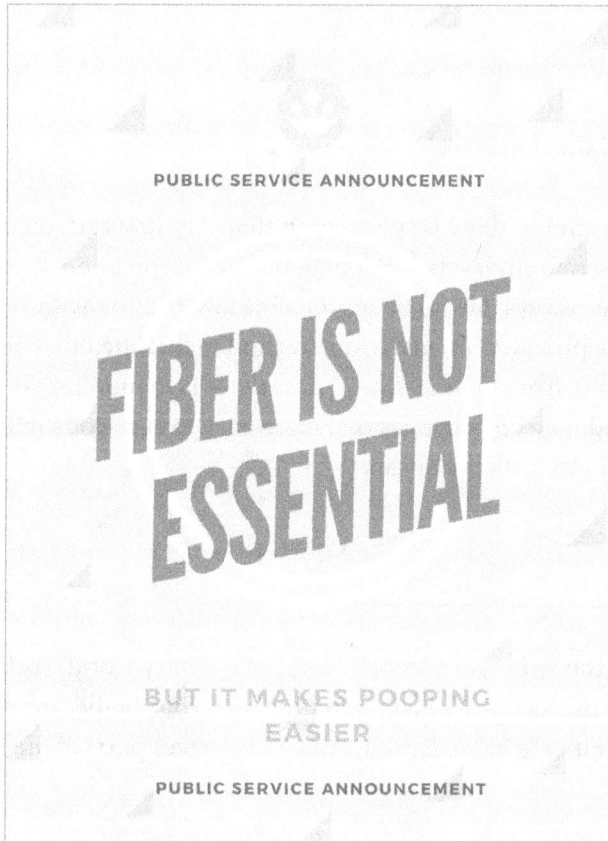

PUBLIC SERVICE ANNOUNCEMENT

FIBER IS NOT ESSENTIAL

BUT IT MAKES POOPING EASIER

PUBLIC SERVICE ANNOUNCEMENT

Fiber has energy. However, I don't recommend tracking these values for the sake of mental sanity. Stick with logging total carbohydrates, and you will come out all right.

Myth-Busting Mermaid:
Net carbs are a marketing ploy to reduce the numbers on the nutrition label.

Food companies determine "net carbs" by subtracting sugar alcohols and fiber. This creates the illusion of lower numbers. Don't fall for their marketing tactics. Total Calories are still important. No matter what voodoo magic they put on the label.

Even though fiber is not essential, target foods with a high amount.

Aim for 30 grams of fiber daily.[27]

Manufacturers routinely add fiber to their products. Beware of your fiber intake dropping, if you reduce the amount of processed foods in your diet. Eat plenty of fruits and veggies to replace any cereals or grains.

A word of caution: If your current intake is far from 25 to 30 grams, proceed slowly. Really, really slowly. Like the tortoise and the hare, slow. Your hind end will thank me for this. Gradually increase the amount of fiber in your diet over a few weeks. Make sure you are drinking plenty of water.

Homework time: Determine the fiber content of your 10 favorite fruits and vegetables.

Alcohol

I don't really want to step in this flaming pile of poo, but I can't get out of this section without mentioning adult beverages. Alcohol has large amounts of energy, registering 7 Calories/gram. Unfortunately, the body considers it a toxin. Consumption of spirits is a deeply personal choice and like many things we discuss, you do you, boo. Just don't forget to track it and any fancy mixers you use.

Micronutrients

Vitamins and minerals are secondary components of our food—the micronutrients. We measure them in milligrams (mg) or micrograms (mcg). The body needs 13 different vitamins. However, there is some debate about which minerals are essential. I have heard cases ranging from 13 to 18, or even more if you are conversing with Kelly from high school selling juice pills.

Micronutrients are responsible for functions in every tissue in the body, including water balance, blood clotting, and bone health. They routinely receive positive press for their importance in the immune system and anti-oxidant capabilities. Anti-oxidant is a swanky word for something that prevents cell and tissue damage. I won't take this opportunity to bog you down with all the details of every single micronutrient. Instead, I'd like to highlight a few common terms that often show up in nutrition landia.

Let's start with vitamins—organic substances made by plants and animals. They can be water soluble and not stored in the body (vitamins B and C), or they are fat soluble and stored in the liver or fat cells (vitamins A, D, E and K). Remember, the body makes vitamin D from cholesterol, when exposed to sunlight.

Minerals are chemical elements (flashback to the periodic table) that living creatures cannot synthesize. They are inorganic, which is just a swanky way to say they come from the earth. Plants do the heavy lifting and get them from the soil. Microorganisms, like bacteria and fungi, process them into complex molecules that animals farther up the food chain use. Also known as, we eat the things that eat the things that steal the things from rocks.

It's easy enough to perform a search on the interwebs to find out what foods contain what micronutrients. But how much do we need? Do we need an entire head of broccoli or just a few Brussel sprouts wrapped in bacon? Thankfully, nutrition scientists have given us a bit of a head start.

Researchers have determined Recommended Daily Allowances (RDA) for micronutrients. If the data is insufficient, they provide Adequate Intake (AI) numbers instead. The problem is that both values suck.

These numbers are the minimum amount not to have disease. For example, the recommendation for vitamin C is not what you need to live yo' best life—it's what you need to not have scurvy. The RDA for vitamin D is almost 10 times less than what researchers think the body needs to reduce the risk of respiratory infection.[28] I'm not advocating guzzling down mass quantities of supplements, but don't give yourself a pat on the back if you are barely meeting "adequate" intake numbers.

Vitamin deficiencies are more common than toxicities.[29] Almost half of the population is not at adequate vitamin D levels. You know what's even worse? Vitamin D deficiency in African Americans may be as high as 80 percent.[30] What about our animal advocates? Plant-based diets require extra care and planning. Pay special attention to both vitamin B and iron. And for grandma? She has a higher probability of being deficient in vitamin B and calcium.[31] Shout out to all my ladies who still have a period. Unfortunately, menstruating females are at a higher risk of iron deficiency. Yeah, girl power.

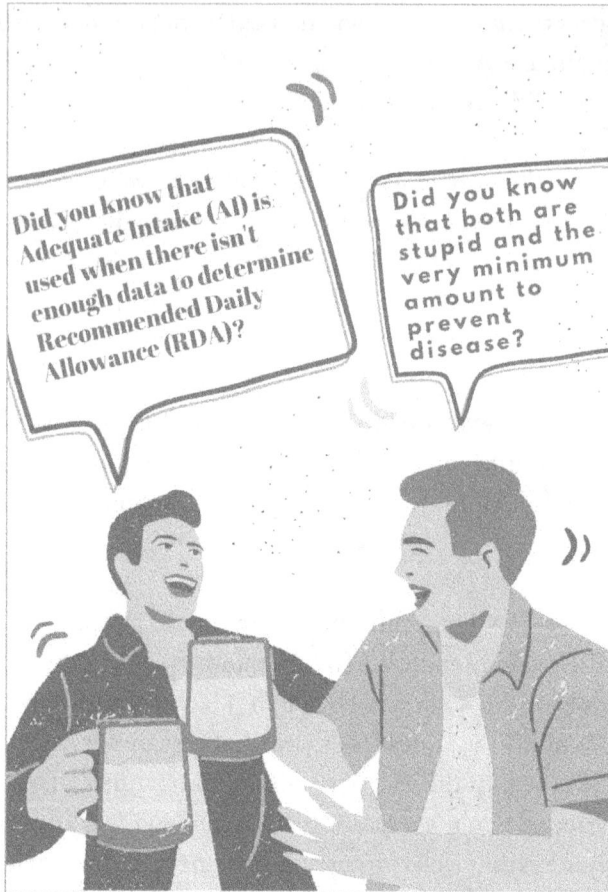

The safest way to get the required amounts of vitamins and minerals is through food. Worried you may have a deficiency? Partner with your primary care provider. There are simple blood tests to determine your numbers. If you supplement, I recommend purchasing from a company with certified third party testing. Stay away from "mega" doses. That money goes straight into the toilet. Or worse, potentially harmful levels build up in your body.

Myth-Busting Mermaid:
Mega dose vitamins are mega piles of poo.

Water

Water is an essential macronutrient. Shocking, right? I did not include it in the macro discussions because it contains no caloric or energy value. I'm only including it here because there will be some troll on the interwebs who points out that I missed it.

How much should you drink? There is actually no consensus, and the 8-cups-a-day recommendation is outdated. A good rule of thumb: drink until you have straw-colored urine. The first deposit of the day is concentrated, so it doesn't count. I could make a case that most of us should drink more, but using the restroom every 2 hours is not the answer either.

---

1. JH Kellogg. *Plain Facts for Old and Young: Embracing the Natural History and Hygiene of Organic Life*. Segner & Condit, 1981.
2. Elango, R and RO Ball. "Protein and amino acid requirements during pregnancy." *Adv Nutr*, 2016 Jul 7 (4): 839-44S.
3. Schoenfeld, BJ and AA Aragon. "How much protein can the body use in a single meal for muscle-building? Implications for daily protein distribution." *J Int Soc Sport Nutr*, 2018 Feb 27 (15):10.
4. Frankenfield, D. "Energy expenditure and protein requirements after traumatic injury." *Nutr Clin Pract*, 2006 Oct 21 (5):430-7.
5. Mettler, F, et al. "Increased protein intake reduces lean body mass loss during weight loss in athletes." *Med Sci Sports Exerc*, 2010 Feb 42 (2): 326-37.
6. Morais, JA, et al. "Protein turnover and requirements in the healthy and frail elderly." *Nutr Health Aging*, 2006 Jul-Aug 10 (4): 272-83.
7. Approximate value based on Dietary Reference Intake (DRI) of 0.36g protein/lb body weight.
8. Mozaffarian, D, et al. "Trans fatty acids and cardiovascular disease." *N Engl J Med*, 2006 Apr 13; 354 (15): 1601-13.
9. Hu, FB, et al. "Diet, lifestyle, and the risk of type 2 diabetes mellitus in women." *N Engl J Med*, 2001 Sep 13; 345 (11): 790-7.
10. de Souza, RK, et al. "Intake of saturated and trans unsaturated fatty acids and risk of all cause mortality, cardiovascular disease, and type 2 diabetes: systematic review and meta-analysis of observational studies." *BMJ*, 2015 Aug 11 (351): h3978.
11. Lambert, CP, et al. "Macronutrient considerations for the sport of bodybuilding." *Sports Med*, 2004; 34 (5): 317-27.
12. Astrup, A, et al. "Saturated Fats and health: a reassessment and proposal for food-based recommendations: JACC stat-of-the-art-review." *J Am Coll Cardiol*, 2020 Aug 18; 76 (7): 844-857.

13. Schwingshacki, L and G Hoffmann. "Monosaturated fatty acids and risk of cardiovascular disease: synopsis of the evidence available from systematic reviews and meta-analysis." *Nutrients*, 2012 Dec 4 (12): 1989-2007.

14. Alpha-linolenic acid, Eicosapentaenoic acid and Docosahexaenoic acid, respectively. I didn't want to muddle up the body of the text with names you need not remember.

15. Mohajeri, M Hasan, et al. "Inadequate supply of vitamins and DHA in the elderly: implications for brain aging and Alzheimer-type dementia." *Nutrition,* 2015 Feb 31 (2): 261-75.

16. Dong, X, et al. Association of dietary Omega-3 and Omega-6 fatty acid intake with cognitive performance in older adults: National Health and Nutrition Examination Survey (NHANES) 2011-2014." *Nutr J*, 2020 Mar 28; 19 (1): 25.

17. Godos, J, et al. "Diet and mental health: review of the recent updates on molecular mechanisms." *Antioxidants (Basel)*, 2020 Apr 9 (4): 346.

18. Ebrahimi, M, et al. "Omega-3 fatty acid supplements improve the cardiovascular risk profile of subjects with metabolic syndrome, including biomarkers of inflammation and auto-immunity." *Act Cardiol*, 2009 Jun 64 (3): 321-7.

19. Custodero, C, et al. "Evidence-based nutritional and pharmacological interventions targeting chronic low-grade inflammation in middle-age and older adults: a systematic review and meta-analysis." *Ageing Res Rev*, 2018 Sep (46): 42-59.

20. Heileson, JL and LK Funderburk. "The effect of fish oil supplementation on the promotion and preservation of lean body mass, strength, and recovery from physiological stress in young, healthy adults: a systemic review." *Nutr Rev*, 2020 Jun 1: nuaa034.

21. More mumbo-jumbo, but included for the sake of completeness. ARA is arachidonic acid.

22. Blasbalg, TL, et al. "Changes in consumption of Omega-3 and Omega-6 fatty acids in the United States during the 20th century." *Am J Clin Nutr*, 2011 May 93 (5): 950-62.

23. Approximate value based on recommended dietary allowance (RDA).

24. Kerksick, CM, et al. "International society of sports nutrition position stand: nutrient timing." *Int Soc Sports Nutr*, 2017 Aug 29 (14): 33.

25. Yabutt, JM, et al. "Emerging roles for serotonin in regulating metabolism: new implications for an ancient molecule." *Endocr Rev*, 2019 Aug 40 (4): 1092-1107.

26. Shabbir, F, et al. "Effect of diet on serotonergic neurotransmission in depression." *Neurochem Int*, 2013 Feb 62 (3): 324-9.

27. Value based on recommendations by the American Heart Association

28. Martineau, AR, et al. "Vitamin D supplementation to prevent acute respiratory tract infections: systemic review and meta-analysis of individual participant data." *BMJ*, 2017 Feb 15 (356): i6583.

29. Blumberg, JB, et al. "Vitamin and mineral intake is inadequate for most Americans: what should we advise patients about supplements?" *J Fam Pract*, 2016 Sept 65 (9 Suppl): S1-S8.

30. Forrest, KYZ and WL Stuhldreher. "Prevalence and correlates of vitamin D deficiency in US adults." *Nutr Res*, 2011 Jan 31 (1): 48-54.

31. Emiroglu, C, et al. "The relationship between nutritional status, anemia and other vitamin deficiencies in the elderly receiving home care." *J Nutr Health Aging*, 2019; 23 (7): 677-82.

2

CALORIES AND SWANKY LAW STUFF

Vending machines kill four times as many people per year as sharks.

D o you want to hear a joke? Okay, here goes... A dung beetle walks into a bar and says, "Excuse me, is this stool taken?" Who doesn't love a good icebreaker poop joke? Not urbane enough for you? How about: Why did the hipster chemist get burned? Because he touched the beaker before it was cool. Get it? Hipster... cool. Not funny? Okay, tough crowd. Let's switch gears. I'd like to tell you about this book I just finished reading. It was about helium, and I couldn't put it down. I kid, I kid. Bear with me for one more. This one applies to the topic at hand. What do you call an acid with an attitude? A-mean-oh acid!

I've always had a fascination with science and was that nerdy kid who wanted to be a chemist instead of a ballerina. Who else geeked out on fruit fly crosses in genetics lab? Or stayed late to make an extra batch of acetaminophen in chemistry class? Did you also complete the bonus problems at the end of the physics chapter? While I like to picture myself in the image of a Hermione Granger, I am a closer resemblance to Velma Dinkley à la Scooby Doo.

Even though I consider these next few sections as thrilling dinner conversation, I realize that many others do not share in my enthusiasm. We will still need to lay a basic scientific foundation to understand how to gain and lose weight. I will simplify a complex process. My aim is to give you enough knowledge to smell the bunk that pervades pop culture weight loss media from a mile away.

∽

Calories
Our first task is to define a calorie. One calorie is the amount of energy (or heat) used to raise the temperature of one gram of water by one degree Celsius. Too scientific for you? Just remember a calorie is energy.

No-Drama Llama Rule:
A calorie is a calorie.

Food and nutrition scientists use a bomb calorimeter to measure the heat from combustion of foods. A calorimeter is just a swanky tool used to determine the energy created when food burns. It records the results in 1,000s of Calories (kcals). Food labels use Calories with a capital "C" to note the amount of energy in a serving of food.

Scientists have determined the amount of Calories in macronutrients for us. Thanks, science. These values are not absolute. However, they are the agreed upon constants in nutrition science, and I use them throughout this book.

Macronutrient Calorie Conventions
1 gram of protein = 4 Calories
1 gram of carbohydrate = 4 Calories
1 gram of fat = 9 Calories
1 gram of alcohol = 7 Calories

Rarely is food in pure macronutrient form. It's more common to eat something that is a mix of 2 or all 3 macronutrients.

For example, meat is a combination of protein and some fat. The percentage of fat in meat determines how lean it is. A chicken breast has less fat than a nice rib-eye cut of steak making it a leaner type of meat.

Tastier meats have higher amounts of fat. I've never craved a baked chicken breast, but there have been times I would have sacrificed a digit for a porterhouse.

When a source claims that not all Calories are equal, they are sensationalizing a food group or macronutrient to fit their dogma.[1, 2, 3] Use your common sense filter and don't fall for the hoopla.

Let me give you an example. Compare a donut that is 300 Calories and a piece of steak that is 300 Calories. They both provide the same amount of energy to the consumer.

However, the macronutrients of steak are more nutritious, require more energy to process, and promote fullness in most individuals.

I'm not advocating eating one type of food over the other; *I'm just pointing out that 300 Calories of energy is 300 Calories of energy.*

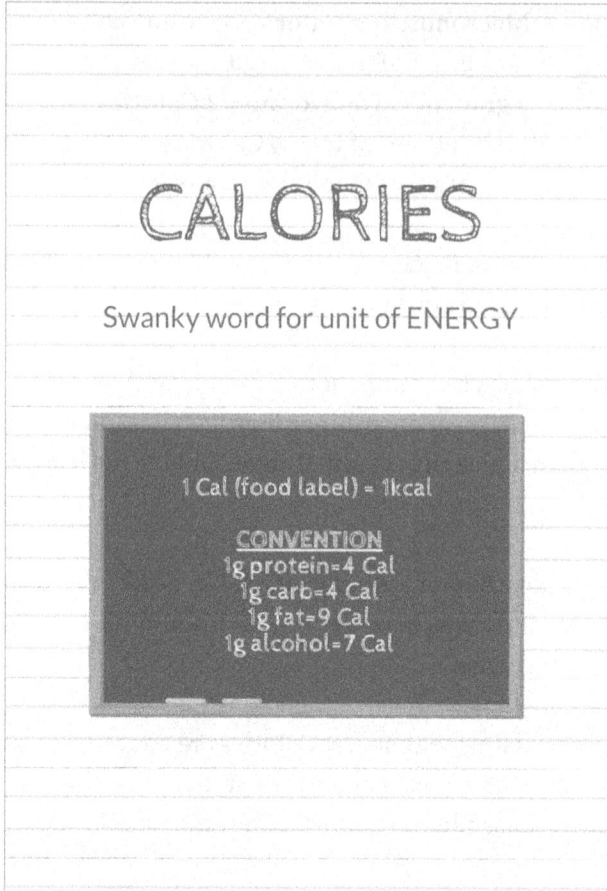

CALORIES

Swanky word for unit of ENERGY

1 Cal (food label) = 1kcal

CONVENTION
1g protein=4 Cal
1g carb=4 Cal
1g fat=9 Cal
1g alcohol=7 Cal

Swanky Law Stuff

Laws in nature are rules to explain repeated observations. They imply a cause-and-effect relationship under certain conditions. If I do "A" to "B" (in a certain environment), then "C" always occurs. This differs from scientific theories, which are interested in "the why." The physical law that applies to weight change is The Law of Conservation of Energy.

The energy of a system is conserved.
It is neither created nor destroyed; energy transfers.

We observe this in an engine. Fuel (energy) goes in and the motor runs (energy out). In an internal combustion engine, like in our vehicles, fuel burns to create heat, and the heat is used to make the wheels on the bus go round and round. This is not a perfect system. Some heat does not transfer as mechanical energy but gets released during the process. Public Service Announcement: Don't touch a motor after running.

Fuel = Heat (given off) + Mechanical Work (heat transferred)

OR

Energy IN = energy OUT

The body digests food and converts it to energy. The fuel is used to power our cells and tissues. Energy is necessary for sustaining life, maintaining an internal temperature, and doing work (like kicking a soccer ball or getting up to pour another glass of wine).

Calories IN = Calories OUT

Energy IN is simple. It is just the food you consume or what you shovel into your donut hole. Energy OUT is where it gets more complex.

Energy IN = food

AND

Energy OUT = genetics, hormones, medicine/medical conditions, exercise and movement, baseline metabolism, internal temperature, energy used for digestion...

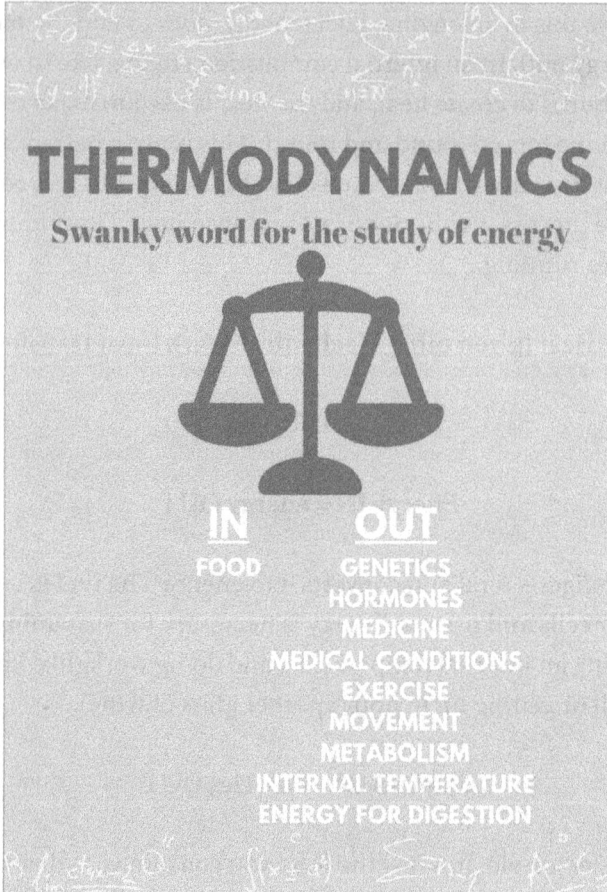

Calories In Calories Out, or CICO in dieting communities, is not calorie counting.

I'll say it louder for those in the back—CICO is not Calorie counting. It is a natural law and is always in play, even if you are not actively tracking.

No-Drama Llama Rule:
CICO is not tracking; it is law.

Fat loss can only occur in a Calorie deficit. Notice that I didn't say weight loss. I'm splitting hairs here, but it's an important distinction.

The number on the scale can change whether you are in a Calorie deficit, Calorie surplus, or maintaining caloric intake. Sadly, it can go in an opposite direction from the one you intended. I will go out on a limb here and assume you are reading this book to learn how to reduce fat, increase muscle mass, or accomplish both. In that case, it's important to stop chasing the number on the scale and focus on body re-composition. Body re-composition is just a swanky term for decreasing fat and increasing muscle.

It is important to pay attention to both sides of the equation. As a diet book, we will look at the energy IN aspect, but I would be remiss if we didn't address the OUT. Everyone can control what goes down the hatch.

Conversely, many things that influence how much energy we spend during the day are out of our control. We cannot change our age, our height, our biological parents, and many medical conditions. Instead, we will focus on the workable items that can help balance the right side of the equation in our favor.

Next, we have some more heavy science-y stuff about food composition. I promise that I won't subject you to any more corny science jokes. In any case, all the good ones Argon.

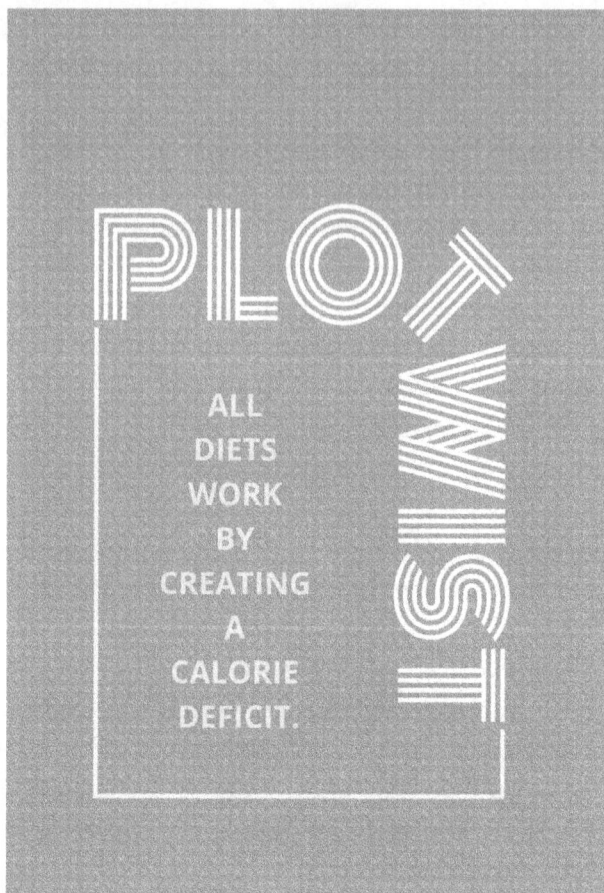

PLOTWIST

ALL
DIETS
WORK
BY
CREATING
A
CALORIE
DEFICIT.

Energy Density and Putting a Bow on It

How do all these nutrient pieces fit together? And what is the best way to determine the energy content of our favorite foods? Will they fit in with our macronutrient goals? Remember, each macronutrient has energy. Also, most of us don't consume pure nutrients. For example, chicken is both protein and fat. Here are two challenges that illustrate these points:

Homework Time: Is it a Protein/Carb/Fat?

1) Find a favorite food in your pantry or refrigerator.

2) Use the nutrition label to determine the total grams of fat, protein, and carbohydrates.

3) Find the serving size and total Calories.

4) Draw a Venn diagram with 3 circles, and place your chosen item in the appropriate spot. New to Venn diagrams? Refer to the image for an example layout.

5) If the serving size is smaller than your palm, then put a star next to it for "energy dense."

> Here's our first example: Skim milk is a combination of protein and carbohydrates. It belongs in the area of the diagram where these 2 overlap. A serving size is 80 Calories for 8 oz, so I would not classify this as an energy-dense food.

> Here's another example for creamy peanut butter: It's a combination of fat, protein, and carbohydrates. Fat is 2x higher than either protein or carbs. Place in the very center of the diagram, where all 3 circles overlap. A serving size is 2 tablespoons for 180 Calories; therefore, I would classify this as a very energy dense food. Mark it with a star.

This is a huge pet peeve of mine. Nuts are a fat with an okay amount of protein. Stop blindly consuming nuts and nut butters and calling them protein!

Myth-Busting Mermaid:
Food companies market peanut butter as a "great" protein source.

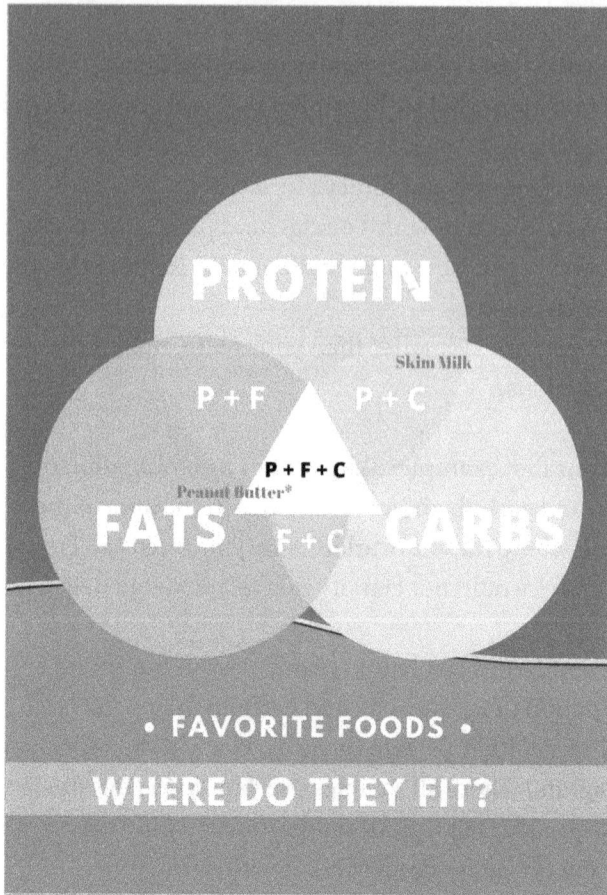

Homework Time: Make a diagram with all of your favorite foods. Yes, there are infographics already available online with all this information. I find it valuable to complete this exercise individually for a few reasons. One, you remember it better if you put pen to paper. Two, you customize the chart with the foods you consume most often. For instance, if you are a vegetarian then there is no reason to hang a chart with types of meat on your fridge. Finally, few of these images contain Calorie content and serving sizes, which is information everyone should have available.

∿

As you progress through this challenge, note two common threads.

Water plays a role in energy density.

For example, 2 cups of grapes are 100 Calories versus 2 cups of raisins, which are approximately 900 Calories.

Foods high in fiber and water are low in energy density.

Eat your fruits and veggies. Here are my favorite high-fiber but low-ish Calorie foods:

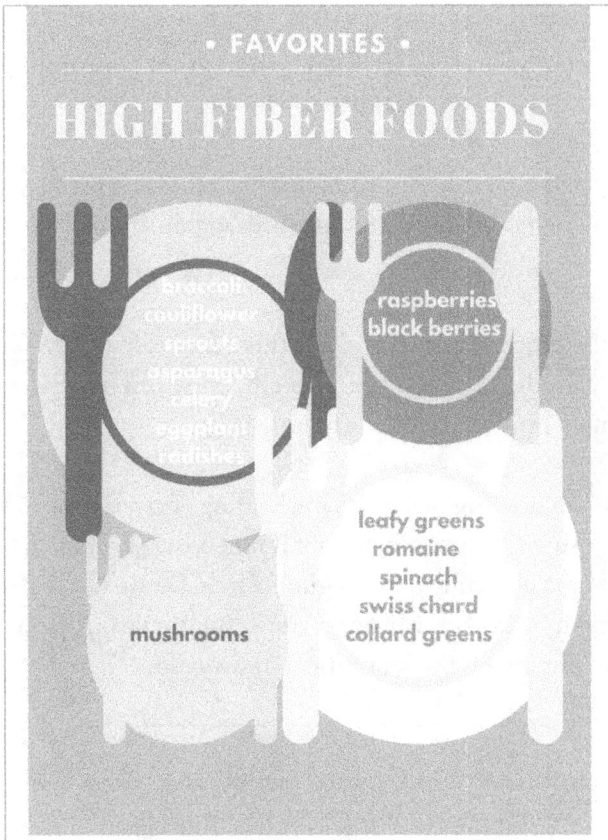

• FAVORITES •

HIGH FIBER FOODS

broccoli
cauliflower
sprouts
asparagus
celery
eggplant
radishes

raspberries
black berries

leafy greens
romaine
spinach
swiss chard
collard greens

mushrooms

After you complete your P/C/F diagram, one very obvious truth stands out.

Oils are the most energy-dense food.

Fats and oils are delicious. I'm not advocating oil-free cooking. That would be the world's saddest diet. However, it is important to keep track of how much you use in the cooking process. This holds true for butter and dressings, which are mostly oil-based.

What about protein? How do you know if something is high in this macronutrient?

Good protein sources are foods with 1 gram of protein per 10 Calories or fewer.

This is my personal rule-of-thumb for protein. Lean meats exceed this ratio, which is why you see gym-bros eating entire flocks of chicken.

When at the grocery store, I will use this quick calculation to figure out if dairy products, processed "protein" bars, and other items are going to meet my macro requirements.

Remember, marketing labels are misleading. Turn the jar over. It's likely not a superb source of protein if it needs a graphic on the front. Also, the sky is blue and water is gluten-free. Do we really need a label telling us that? Nopety, nope, nope. But that won't stop companies from jumping on the latest diet bandwagon.

---

1. Wycherley, TP, et al. "Effects of energy-restricted high-protein, low-fat compared with standard-protein, low-fat diets: a meta-analysis of randomized controlled trials." *Am J Clin Nutr*, 2012 Dec 96 (6): 1281-98.

2. de Souza, RJ, et al. "Effects of weight-loss diets differing in fat, protein, and carbohydrate on fat mass, lean mass, visceral adipose tissue, and hepatic fat: results from the POUNDS LOST trial." *Am J Clin Nutr*, 2012 Mar 95 (3): 614-25.

3. Johnston, CS, et al. "Ketogenic low-carbohydrate diets have no metabolic advantage over nonketogenic low-carbohydrate diets." *AM J Clin Nutr*, 2006 May 83 (5): 1055-61.

ALL ABOUT THE BENJAMINS—ENERGY AS CURRENCY

Chicken soup was considered an aphrodisiac in the middle ages.

The growth of crystals is a natural process when molecules precipitate out of a solution. Precipitate is just a swanky word for something solid separating from its liquid form. This occurs quickly, like with the formation of ice. Or it can occur more slowly. Diamonds take millennia to form. The process starts when the first molecules gather, forming a nucleus. Nucleus is a swanky word for the center of an object. More and more particles combine, creating a seed crystal. This structure serves as a foundation for branching. Tiny imperfections in the original nucleus amplify, creating unique shapes.

We find examples of crystallization in the kitchen. Do you have an old jar of honey? Remove the cap, and you will probably discover tiny crystals that have formed around the lid. Want to speed up this process? Place the jar in the fridge for two days. The cooler temperature inside will cause more molecules to precipitate. This happens in nature, too.

Let's look at the process for making honey. Once the bellies of the forager bees are full of nectar from flowers, they make the return trip back to the hive and regurgitate the contents to worker bees. Seriously, the bees vomit nectar from their honey stomach. The worker bees then pass the nectar around to each other until it breaks down. They place the honey in individual cells of the comb, and house bees furiously fan their wings, generating heat to evaporate out most of the water. Wax caps the cells, sealing it for later use during the winter months. When the cell is first filled, the honey is liquid. Over time, crystals develop, following the same process as ice or diamonds.

I don't have a hive of workers to make honey, but last spring I created sugar glass in the kitchen with my kiddos. Much to my dismay, they didn't appreciate the science behind the crystallization process. All four wanted more candy-making and less science talk. The best part? When we stirred the super-heated mixture and removed the spoon, it revealed a dingle-berry of sugar. Their description, not mine.

Want to know what happens when super-heated sugar spins around at dizzying speeds and travels through very tiny holes? You get the airy stuff of carnival dreams—cotton candy. The sugar cools too rapidly to allow the formation of crystals. Instead, amorphous fibers form. Amorphous is just a swanky word for something without a defined shape, like clouds. Misters John Wharton and William Morrison unveiled this tasty treat at the 1904 World's Fair in St. Louis. It successfully debuted under the name of Fairy Floss. Fitting, considering it was the invention of a candy maker and dentist.

~

Energy Storage in the Body

You may have already heard the nectar-to-honey story. Honeybees forage all season and build up their honey supplies. This helps them overwinter when vegetation is scarce, but did you know that pollen is actually the preferred food source of bees? Along with nectar and water, it provides all the protein, fats, and micronutrients that a bee diet requires. Bees prefer to dine on pollen because making honey is a metric crap ton of work.

Unlike our flying friends, we do not store energy in combs. The human body has an entirely different way to store energy. Here is an analogy that might help. Think of fuel from food as money. Let's treat it as currency. For our purposes,

Glucose = Cash in your wallet

AND

Glycogen = Cash under your mattress

AND

Fat = Local bank account

AND

Protein = Loan from friends and family

I realize this analogy is outdated, as most of us rely on plastic. However, the intangibility of credit cards doesn't lend itself to our story. Play along.

Glucose in your blood (from carbs) travels around the body to supply tissues for immediate use. This is the cash in your wallet.

The body stores any extra glucose by forming glycogen in the liver and muscle tissue. Remember, glycogen is a long strand of linked glucose molecules. Think of it as the cash you store under your mattress, for when you don't want to run to the ATM.

In the body, fat cells act as a savings account of energy. We dip into our "savings account," after depleting glycogen. This keeps the body running until you eat your next meal. Similar to money accounts, you make deposits when there is an abundance of energy from food.

What happens when you run low on funds? One solution is to get a loan from a family member or friend. If it floats you until your next paycheck, then you gotta do what you gotta do.

Your body does not prefer to burn protein as fuel, but it will under duress. For prolonged time between meals, the body breaks down lean muscle and organ tissue for survival. In developed countries, we commonly observe this in elderly individuals, in patients ravaged by illness, and in very lean athletes who are cutting for weight-controlled competition.

What if you are working overtime at your primary gig, plus your side hustle is doing well? In real life, rolling in the Benjamins is not an awful place to be. For our analogy, this is when you consume more Calories than the body needs at the moment.

Honestly, the body doesn't really have much of a problem with it either. Its bank account, fat tissue, is virtually unlimited. The body is happy to keep squirreling away the excess fuel in the off chance the future may hold a scarcity of food.

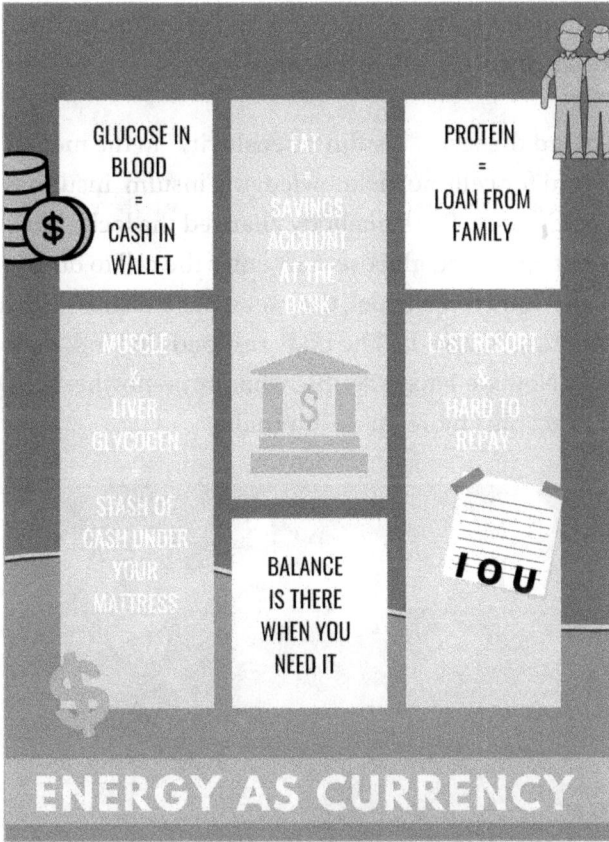

GLUCOSE IN BLOOD = CASH IN WALLET

FAT = SAVINGS ACCOUNT AT THE BANK

PROTEIN = LOAN FROM FAMILY

MUSCLE & LIVER GLYCOGEN = STASH OF CASH UNDER YOUR MATTRESS

LAST RESORT & HARD TO REPAY

BALANCE IS THERE WHEN YOU NEED IT

I O U

ENERGY AS CURRENCY

Keeping with the money analogy, there is one important player in all of this—insulin.

Think of insulin as the body's financial advisor.

After a meal, insulin directs the levels of glucose in the blood (cash in wallet), promotes the formation of glycogen in liver and muscle (cash under mattress), increases fat storage (deposits in bank), and inhibits muscle wasting (doesn't ask The Fam for a loan). Phew, that's some heavy hitting.

Almost all cells in the body respond to insulin. It is a protein molecule that acts like a key and opens a channel in cell membranes.

Imagine a tunnel into the cell blocked by a gate. Insulin opens the gate, allowing glucose to enter the cell.

Have you heard the term "insulin insensitivity" in the media? It's just a swanky word for cells not acknowledging insulin. Insulin is knocking on the gate. But somebody changed the locks. Now, the door does not open, and glucose can't enter the cell to do all the things. If cells don't receive fuel, they send out a distress signal, telling the body they are "starved." The body responds in kind, making its own glucose. Now we have a double whammy—nowhere for glucose from food to go, plus more made internally.

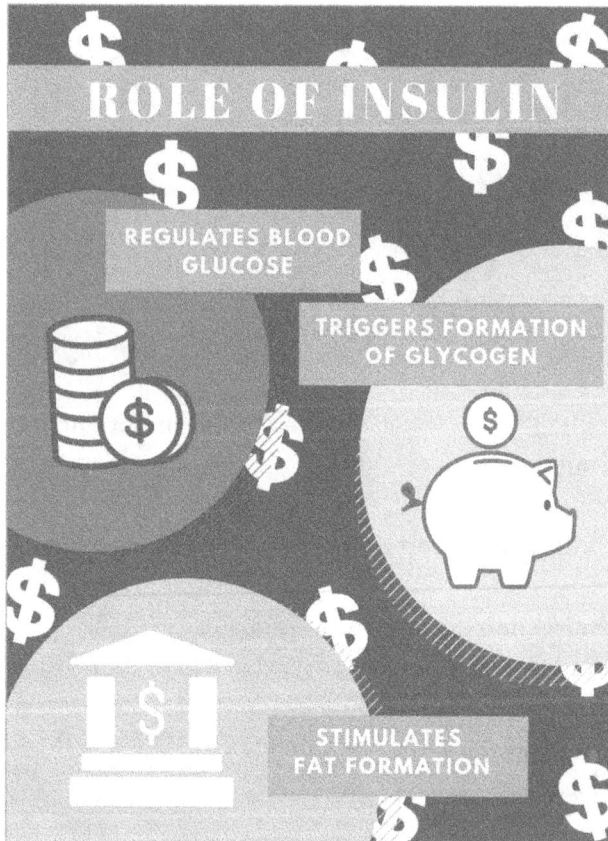

ROLE OF INSULIN

REGULATES BLOOD GLUCOSE

TRIGGERS FORMATION OF GLYCOGEN

STIMULATES FAT FORMATION

Fat Storage and Dieting
Too long? Don't want to read? Our fat suit is the energy storage location for lipids we consume.

The longer version—adipose tissue is a complex organ. Adipose is just a swanky word for fat. There are two types of fat tissue in the body. We characterize each by their unique cells and functions.

White adipose tissue (WAT) is our largest energy reserve. It also insulates and provides a cushion for our organs. This is our main storage depot for triglycerides from food and excess glucose.

Low-carb zealots will harp and harp on this last point. Yes, the body converts excess carbs to glucose and stores them as fat. BUT. ALL. EXCESS. CALORIES. ARE. CONVERTED. AND. STORED. IN. FAT. CELLS. Don't you hate it when caps lock gets stuck?

No-Drama Llama Rule:
We store all excess Calories as fat, not just carbs.

On a side note, the body keeps a small amount of triglycerides in muscle for fuel. That's super-duper great for those muscle fibers, but we don't consider it a large energy reserve.

Did you know that our body's fat is not *just* an energy silo or winter parka? Today, scientists classify WAT as an endocrine organ. Endocrine is a swanky word for something that releases hormones.

Most notability, WAT produces the hormone leptin. Often referred to as the "satiety hormone," leptin tells your brain that your fat suit is big enough. As a result, the brain suppresses your hunger.

Leptin is the satiety hormone. Our fat makes Leptin.

Here's another fun fact. Scientists discovered a link between WAT and other hormone production. For example, the last step for making estrogen requires an enzyme produced by fat cells. Hardly the inanimate, gelatinous blob we once thought, eh?

～

Brown adipose tissue (BAT) is unique and classified separately from white. It plays an important role in internal temperature regulation for newborns and infants. Scientists label brown fat as "good fat" because it uses energy to perform its job. You read that correctly. Your fat uses fuel, too.

We find brown fat near the shoulder blades and neck. It generates heat in response to cold exposure. Recall, our body uses Calories to stay warm. There is a higher percentage of BAT in children and adolescents, compared to adults. Scientists associate its activation during puberty with less weight gain and more muscle mass during those tortuous years.[1]

Adults have BAT, too, just not as much as infants and adolescents. We can increase our volume of BAT with exercise, adequate sleep, and cold exposure.[2] Who doesn't want more fat that burns Calories? In fact, the browning of WAT is an important area under study for obesity therapy.[3, 4, 5] Browning is a swanky, but very descriptive, term for the conversion of WAT to BAT in response to cold exposure.

So how does fat respond when dieting? We use triglycerides, stored in fat, for fuel. This causes a decrease in the overall size of the individual cells. Straightforward, right? Unfortunately for some individuals, the body then signals slower turnover (or death) of fat cells!

Picture this. You successfully lose those stubborn extra pounds, and your fat cells shrink. Sweet! However, as a protection against prolonged starvation, there is an increase in the number of fat cells in that same area. When you fall off the diet wagon, the fat cells, both old and new, all return to their original size. The problem? Now you have more in the same amount of space. This is a proposed mechanism for obesity, especially as it relates to weight gain from Yo-Yo dieting.[6, 7]

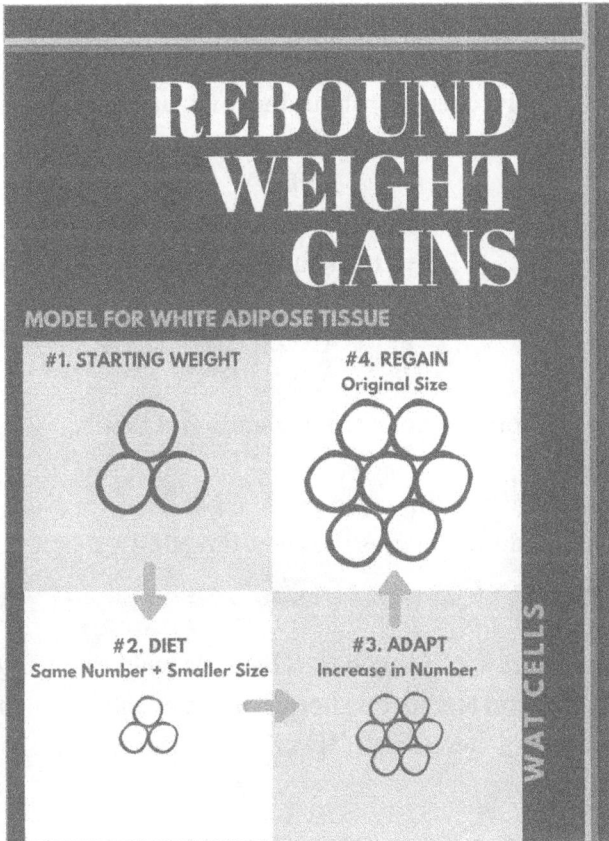

REBOUND WEIGHT GAINS

MODEL FOR WHITE ADIPOSE TISSUE

#1. STARTING WEIGHT

#4. REGAIN
Original Size

#2. DIET
Same Number + Smaller Size

#3. ADAPT
Increase in Number

WAT CELLS

Understanding energy storage in the body will help you weed through the drivel in nutrition media. Don't fall for diet propaganda claiming carbohydrates are the devil. Correctly, when we consume too many, the body stores the excess as fat. You know what else we store as fat if consumed in excess—fat. Also, the body converts excess protein to glucose and, more rarely, fat. Humans store any excess energy shoved down our pieholes as fat.

How Energy Is Used

Let's switch gears and look at the how our body uses energy. Returning to our currency analogy, we have

Glucose = Cash in your wallet

AND

Glycogen = Cash under your mattress

AND

Fat = Local bank account

AND

Protein = Loan from friends and family

After we fill our bellies, energy is abundant and easy to use. This is insulin's time to shine. He runs the show directing resources throughout the body.

Between meals, it's a different story. There is a new sheriff in town— glucagon. Glucagon is a peptide hormone secreted by the pancreas when blood glucose levels drop. He's the boss when the cash in your wallet gets too low.

Side Note: The body also secretes glucagon in response to stress or "stimulation." Ask any Type I diabetic what happens when they are excited.

Think of Glucagon as the body's debt management specialist.

Glucagon is the counterpart to insulin. Its immediate task is to raise blood glucose levels by dipping into the body's glycogen stores.

Glycogen strands in liver and skeletal muscle will sustain energy levels for approximately 12-18 hours, less if there is strenuous activity.

This time frame works well for our daily lives, since most of us would eat within this window. For our model, the money you hid under the mattress will refill your wallet so you can go about your day.

What if that runs out, too? Then it's time for a trip to the bank (fat storage). Glucagon directs adipose tissue to stop storing fatty acids and to increase their circulation in the blood.

This system works well by design. A lot of cells in the body burn fatty acids as fuel. For the handful who require glucose, glucagon stimulates gluconeogenesis in the liver. This produces a small amount to stabilize blood sugar levels and provide enough energy for those cells.

At the end of the line, the body can break down protein from muscle and other organs for energy use. This is our friends and family loan. It works, but it's not ideal.

As our bodies continue along the spectrum from fasting to starvation, this breakdown speeds up. It occurs more rapidly in lean individuals, those with a low fat bank account. That's why it is so important for lean folks to have sufficient protein intake, especially if they are consuming fewer Calories than they are burning.

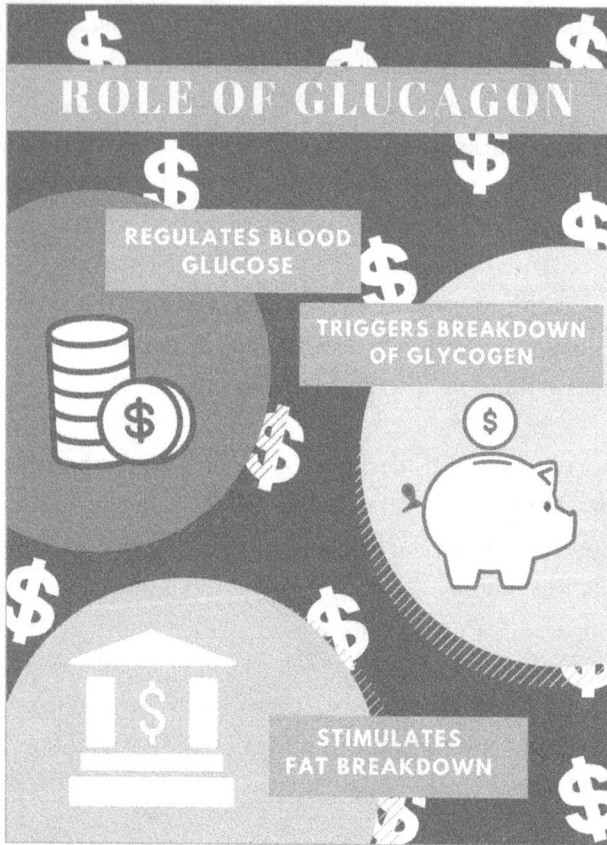

ROLE OF GLUCAGON

REGULATES BLOOD GLUCOSE

TRIGGERS BREAKDOWN OF GLYCOGEN

STIMULATES FAT BREAKDOWN

The energy-as-currency model is not linear. The body doesn't use glucose from blood. Then stops and switches off to glycogen. It doesn't wait until glycogen stores are low to dip into fat. I laid it out that way for teaching.

These processes run simultaneously. For example, the brain likes glucose. It may burn that as fuel, whereas our muscles use fatty acids.

Tissues can use different fuel sources. Muscle likes fatty acids. But when conditions change (i.e. intense exercise), they switch to glucose for some fast energy.

Adipose tissue uses fatty acids. Hey, it's right there. Except right after a meal when it uses glucose. Our kidneys and liver mainly use fatty acids, but red blood cells and retinal cells in your eye use glucose because they lack the machinery to burn lipids.

Cellular Exchange and Brain Fuel
In my simplification of energy storage and use, I glossed over complex biochemical processes. The cycles all have fancy names and haunt the dreams of biochemistry students. They are something you learn for a test and then unlearn 5 minutes after. The information is easily accessible, so if you want to dive into that barrel of monkeys, go forth and enjoy the circus.

However, we need to address how individual cells use energy.

Cells cannot use glucose and fatty acids directly. They must exchange our cash for a different tender. The ultimate currency of the cell is adenosine triphosphate (ATP). Here is our yellow brick road:

We digest macronutrients from food.
(Protein to amino acids)
(Carbohydrates to glucose)
(Fat to triglycerides)

THEN

The building blocks circulate in the blood for use as fuel.

THEN

Individual cells convert these units to ATP.

Let's look at where in the cell this occurs and some common terms thrown around in nutrition media.

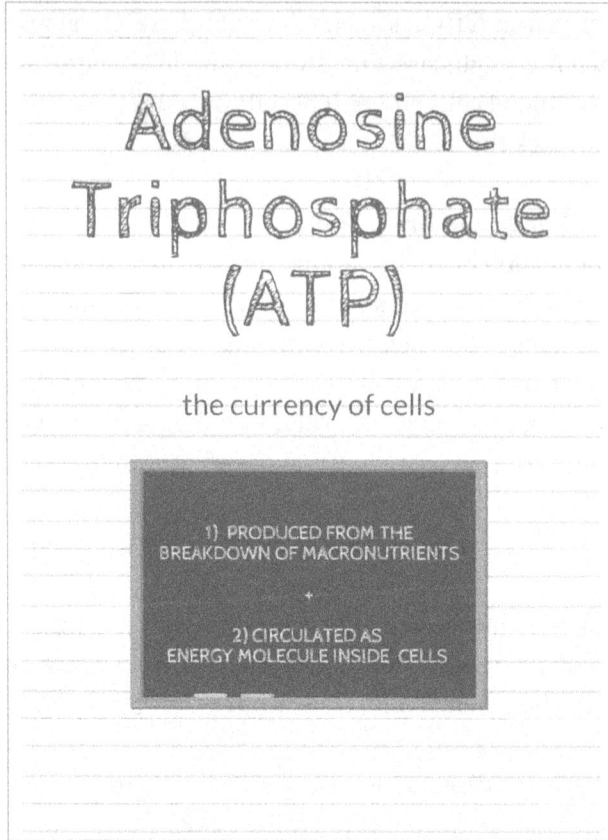

Adenosine Triphosphate (ATP)

the currency of cells

1) PRODUCED FROM THE
BREAKDOWN OF MACRONUTRIENTS

+

2) CIRCULATED AS
ENERGY MOLECULE INSIDE CELLS

For glucose, the first part of the process takes place in the cell's cytoplasm. Cytoplasm is just a swanky work for the gel-like matrix or filling of a cell. The breakdown of glucose in this area occurs without the use of oxygen, or under *anaerobic* conditions.

We shuttle lipids, amino acids, and glucose by-products into the mitochondria. Mitochondria is just a swanky name for the power plants of the cell. They convert these molecules into ATP. These little energy stations provide most of the fuel for the cell to live its best life. This process is a*erobic,* occurring in the presence of oxygen.

Of note, the aerobic pathway generates way more ATP than its anaerobic counterpart.

~

We need to address one last topic in our food-as-currency model. As mentioned before, carbohydrates are not an essential macronutrient. What happens when we remove or restrict them in our diet? And not just for a meal or two. How does the body respond, and how does energy use differ under these conditions? And just what in the heck is *ketosis*?

The ketosis story starts when the body has depleted all of its glycogen stores. Recall, glucagon swoops in and signals the body to create its own glucose molecules via gluconeogenesis.

Why is this last point important? One, there are cells in the body that don't have mitochondria and cannot burn anything other than glucose as fuel. We would like to keep those guys afloat. And two, the brain cannot burn fatty acids as fuel. Not because neurons in the brain lack mitochondria, but because the blood vessels that supply the central nervous system (the brain, spinal cord, and optic nerve) are very, very picky about what they "let through" to the neurons. The blood-brain barrier is just a swanky word for the protective border formed by the walls of those blood vessels. Fatty acids are too large to sneak past this barrier.

The body's defense mechanism against low-carb intake is ketosis. Ketosis is just a swanky word for the formation of ketone bodies. Made in the liver from fatty acids, these molecules are small enough to cross the blood-brain barrier, where neurons use them as fuel. It takes a few weeks for the brain to adapt to using ketones for energy. During that time, most folks experience brain fog—headaches, dizziness, fatigue, and insomnia.

From a fat loss perspective, ketosis sounds intriguing, right? Who doesn't want to burn fat for fuel?

Unfortunately, the Keto Diet still follows the Laws of Thermodynamics. If you are consuming excess Calories, the body will store them.

At the time of this writing, this diet is still all the rage. Yes, I've tried it and no, I'm not a fan for a few reasons. One, my hobbies include explosive, athletic movements; carbohydrates are necessary for optimal performance. Two, I find it very difficult to eat the combination of macronutrients to sustain ketosis long-term. Notice I said, ketosis, not low-carb. A diet low in carbohydrates does not mean your body is in ketosis. Finally, I try to avoid diets that eliminate an entire macronutrient.

Myth-Busting Mermaid:
You can still store fat, while burning mainly fat as fuel.

---

1. Gilsanz, V, et al. "Relevance of brown adipose tissue in infancy and adolescence." *Pediatr Res*, 2013 Jan 73 (1): 3-9.
2. Cohen, P and BM Spiegelman. "Brown and beige fat: molecular parts of a thermogenic machine." *Diabetes*, 2015; 64: 2346-51.
3. Kaisanlahti, A and T Glumoff. "Browning of white fat: agents and implications for beige adipose tissue to type 2 diabetes." *J Physiol Biochem*, 2019 Feb 75 (1): 1-10.
4. Thoonen, R, et al. "Brown adipose tissue: the heat is on the heart." *AM J Physiol Heart Circ Physiol*, 2016 Jun 1; 310 (11): H1592-1605.
5. Kurylowicz, A and M Puzianowska-Kuznicka. "Induction of adipose tissue browning as a strategy to combat obesity." *Int J Mol Sci*, 2020 Sep 21 (17): 6241.
6. Shin, S, et al. "Adipose stem cells in obesity: challenges and opportunities." *Biosci Rep*, 2020 Jun 26; 40 (6): BSR20194076.
7. Engin, A. "Fat cell and fatty acid turnover in obesity." *Adv Exp Med Biol*, 2017; 906: 135-60.

4

TOTAL ENERGY EXPENDITURE

A Twinkie has 37 ingredients.

I magine the evolutionary drive necessary to fly 6 miles in search of a home to lay your eggs. Even when you are no bigger than the size of an eyelash. Upon arrival, instead of a welcoming sight of big, bright petals, nature requires you to use your sense of smell to find hidden flowers inside of hollow balls on a tree. You read that correctly. I said, "laying eggs in tree balls."

Once inside, you squeeze through a passage to reach the center, but it's so small your wings and antennae rip off. You deposit pollen from your birth home along the way and lay eggs fertilized by your biological brother. If you have chosen well, the ripening fruit will not only protect your offspring, it will also graciously dissolve your dead carcass.

Thus is the life cycle of a queen fig wasp. Don't shed a tear for these harrowing females. Their male counterparts have it worse. After hatching and mating with their siblings, their sole purpose in life is to burrow tunnels through the fig fruit as an escape route for their sisters to fly out in search of a new hatching grounds. So they may continue this mutually beneficial arrangement of tree and insect.

Choke on your Fig Newtons? Wondering how many grams of insect protein you've eaten? Better yet, how can we make a side hustle out of selling figs by marketing them as a substantial source of protein, without informing the public about its source? Chances are you've consumed fruit from a commercially cultivated fig tree—one that is sterile, seedless, and bred to not require pollination by the fig wasp. For the ones with seeds, just don't look too closely.

~

The Energy Balancing Act

There is an energy balance between growth, survival, and reproduction. Some organisms grow large whereas others remain small. Certain animals reproduce quickly whereas others only make a few crotch goblins. In nature, many creatures trade longer life spans in favor of rapid growth.

The fig wasp remains small, makes some crazy sacrifices, and uses most of its energy for reproduction. Contrast that to humans, who spend many years just growing. And growing and maybe making a baby or two. No, I'm not your Aunt Sheila asking when you are starting a family. You keep all that extra energy and funnel it into looking and feeling fabulous.

We allocate energy for GROWTH, SURVIVAL, or REPRODUCTION.

Keep this in mind as we break down the energy OUT side of the equation into tiny details. Don't get lost in the weeds. Our bodies want to grow bigger, wake up each morning, and make mini-mes. Thankfully, our giant human brains allow for *some* conscious choice on how we use our Calories. Let's return to our energy equation from earlier.

Calories IN = Calories OUT

Calories IN is the food we consume. Calories OUT is our TOTAL ENERGY EXPENDITURE (TEE). This changes our equation slightly.

Calories IN = TEE

Who's ready for some more acronym funsies? Here we go. We divide TEE into four buckets.

Basal Metabolic Rate (BMR) is our first and largest bucket. Many refer to BMR as our metabolism. Metabolism is just a swanky word for complex chemical reactions inside our bodies that keep us alive. It's the bare minimum to keep the lights on (e.g. keep organs functioning).

Our next bucket is the Thermic Effect of Food (TEF). Digesting food requires energy. Chewing, absorbing, and pooping are not Calorie-free.

Activity and movement also require energy. Jumping around the living room on one foot after stepping on a Lego. Raising a wine glass to our lips. Shouting at our kids to pick up their socks. These actions require fuel. We label this bucket Thermic Effect of Activity or TEA.

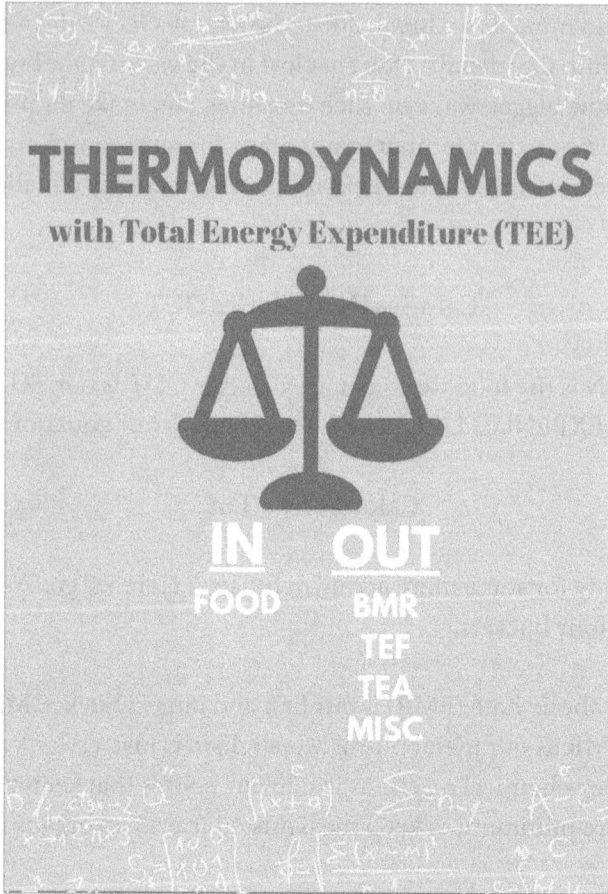

Everything else gets filed under the miscellaneous column. I won't get points in originality for naming things, but you get the drift.

As promised, here is our acronym vomit.

$$TEE = BMR + TEF + TEA + MISC$$

It's time to dive further down into each bucket.

Basal Metabolic Rate

Basal metabolic rate is the amount of energy the body uses just to exist. It requires fuel for breathing, pumping blood, etc. BMR comprises a whopping 60-75% of total calorie expenditure for non-athletes. It's weird to think laying in bed all day, just chilling, burns more Calories than an intense round of exercise. This is the elephant in the equation and the largest component of the energy OUT formula.

Our metabolic rate depends on our biological sex. Males have a higher BMR than females, even if you equate scale weight.

BMR also depends on age, declining 1-2% every decade. This starts in your 20s.

While age and biological sex are out of our control, we can alter our total lean body mass. You may not grow an extra liver or two, but increasing the amount of skeletal muscle on your frame will help increase BMR. Why? Skeletal muscle is very expensive tissue. Your body must use a lot of energy to maintain it.

Age, biological sex, and lean body mass affect BMR.

Side Note: You may find Basal Metabolic Rate used interchangeably with Resting Metabolic Rate (RMR). BMR is more accurate, so I will stick with it for our purposes.

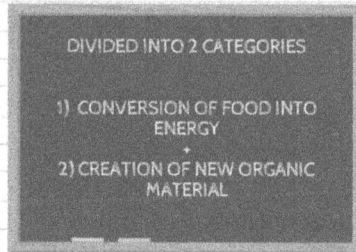

METABOLISM

complex chemical reactions necessary for maintenance of life

DIVIDED INTO 2 CATEGORIES

1) CONVERSION OF FOOD INTO ENERGY
+
2) CREATION OF NEW ORGANIC MATERIAL

Thermic Effect of Food

Breaking down food requires energy. Different macronutrients require different amounts of fuel to process them into usable components. Protein is our gas guzzler. It needs the highest amount of Calories to digest and repackage. Carbohydrates are like mid-level sedans. Some are good on fuel requirements, whereas others need more energy to get the job done. The more complex, longer chain carbohydrates require more energy to breakdown than their simple, short-chain counterparts. Fat from food is like an Italian moped. It's ready to go with a minimal amount of fuel. Here's how the numbers breakdown:

Protein = 20-30% of Calories for processing
Carbohydrates = 5-15% of Calories for processing
Fat = 2-3% of Calories for processing

Since meals are usually a mix of protein, carbs, and fat, I prefer to use a standard of 10% in the TEE equation.

Thermic Effect of Activity
It doesn't require a leap of faith to acknowledge movement requires fuel. Of the components in the total energy equation, this is the most variable between individuals. For someone who is sedentary, TEA might contribute 10% to the Calories OUT side of the equation. On the other end of the spectrum, athletes may use over 50% of their total energy requirements to meet the demands of their sport. There are 4 rules to follow when discussing TEA.

RULE #1: Don't exercise to eat.

This sets up an unhealthy relationship with food. We should not use movement or exercise as a tool to punish consumption of high Calorie items. Everyone must eat to survive, but this mindset is too close to assigning morality to food. Plus, the numbers aren't in your favor. Running a mile and a half to burn a Twinkie is not my idea of a fun time. We also know this rule as, "you can't outtrain a poor diet."

RULE #2: Leave out TEA when calculating Calorie goals.

The amount of Calories burned when exercising is very hard to calculate.

One, machines and fitness trackers usually overestimate the amount of energy burned during a workout. Sad, but true. Repeat after me. "I will not eat as many Calories as my smartwatch says I'm burning."

Two, there is no standard amount of energy assigned for a movement, even for the same individual. For instance, let's say I'm starting a couch-to-5K program, out-of-shape and 20lbs overweight. In theory, my breathing should improve over time, and I may even haul less body weight around the further along I am in the program. The amount of energy I have to use to "not die" on that very first mile is way higher than what I needs a few months later.

Following an exercise program? Great. Have a workout partner you don't flake out on most days. Super. Even on a set schedule, your amount of movement varies daily. This brings us to our third point. It's crazy talk to recalculate our Calories every single day to account for this variation.

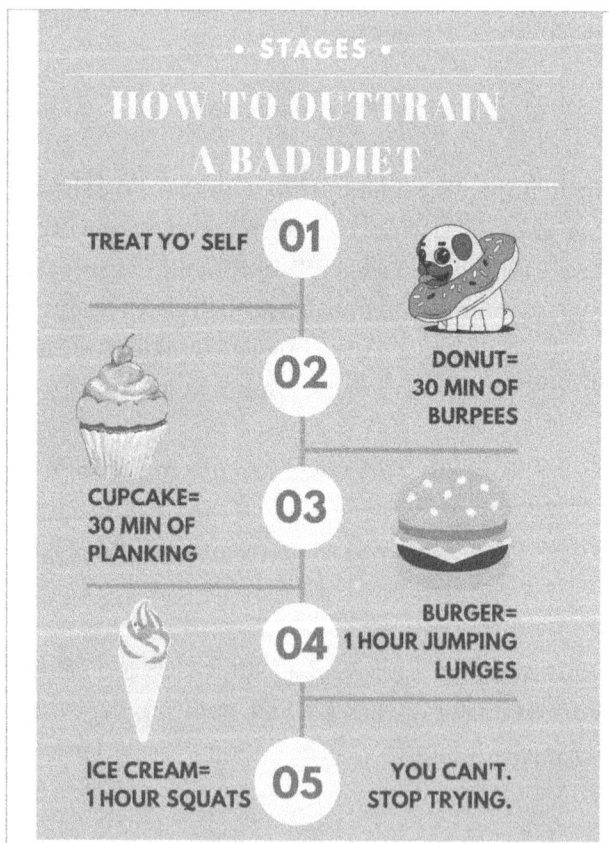

• STAGES •

HOW TO OUTTRAIN A BAD DIET

TREAT YO' SELF **01**

02   DONUT=
30 MIN OF
BURPEES

CUPCAKE=
30 MIN OF
PLANKING   **03**

04   BURGER=
1 HOUR JUMPING
LUNGES

ICE CREAM=
1 HOUR SQUATS   **05**   YOU CAN'T.
STOP TRYING.

RULE #3: Leave out EPOC when calculating Calorie goals.

There is a phenomenon known as Excess Post-Exercise Oxygen Consumption (EPOC). EPOC is just a swanky phrase for the amount of energy required for your body to return to baseline after a hard training session. This is analogous to a car engine taking extra time to cool off after a long road trip. The intensity of training, more than the duration, is the biggest influence on EPOC.[1]

Myth-Busting Mermaid:
EPOC is a thing, but gyms exaggerate its effect to get you into boot camp classes.

Immediately after a workout, your body needs to cool off, get some more oxygen in the ole lungs, and replace ATP stores. Later, it also has to replenish glycogen and repair skeletal muscle damage. All of this increases BMR in the day or two after an intense workout. Cool beans, right?

Straight talk. Calculating EPOC is difficult. Just leave it out of the equation.

Rule #4: Find something you love, or just walk until you do.

What if I told you that to lose weight and keep it off, all you had to do is swim across a lake every morning? It wouldn't be an enormous lake, just large enough that a trip across and back would take maybe 20 or 30 minutes. In our magical tale, I would even ensure the temperature of the water is tolerable year-round and there were no creepy crawlies to nibble at your toes.

Would you do it? How many days in a row do you think you would last? How would you plan for vacations? Out of town work schedules? Illnesses? I'm sure in the beginning, when motivation is high and results are immediate, it wouldn't be that hard to continue. What do you think would happen when you reach your goal weight or ideal body composition? How much harder do you think it would be to get up every morning and take that swim? Day in and day out.

Picture this lake analogy when starting an exercise program. Are you doing something you love or at least, don't hate? CONSISTENCY is key when adding exercise to your schedule. There are endless possibilities from which to choose, so why not pick one that you will stick with even when tired, or busy, or not in the mood? And who says you have to do just one?

Make a goal, enjoy the journey, crush it, and repeat. Or choose a new goal.

I'm more comfortable with the science-y stuff than this rah, rah go-team monologue. You get the point. Don't know where to start? Just put in the steps until you do. That's not a euphemism for something else. Literally, walk and increase your daily step count.

Miscellaneous
This is the catchall category. I'm going to randomly assign a value of 5 percent for this bucket, mainly because it works with my maths. In reality, it should not account for much of the total Calories OUT for the day.

The two major components of this group are cold adaptation and non-exercise activity thermogenesis, or NEAT. Technically, regulation of internal temperature more closely aligns with BMR. I want to tease it out here because under certain circumstances it can have a higher energy demand than normal.

Mostly, in developed countries, we live a soft life. Running from one temperature-controlled box to another, from our homes to our cars to our workplace or retail shops. Compare that existence to someone whose occupation requires him or her to be out in the elements year-round. Or children who still have outdoor recess and physical education, those lucky punks.

Shivering burns energy.

The other element that can have a measurable impact on energy expenditure is NEAT, basically any movement you didn't plan.

My mother would call this fidgeting or futzing around the house. There is a genetic component to unintentional finger drumming or leg shaking. You know who you are. Beware, experts will succumb to a Twitter feud over what makes up NEAT. Many will count walking or purposely increasing step counts in this category, whereas others proclaim that we *plan* the morning stroll with the pooch, so it should fall under TEA. Who gives a flying rat's tookus? There are bigger issues to debate in the Twitter-verse.

∿

THERE IS A SAYING IN MEDICINE: "When you hear hoofbeats, look for horses, not zebras." Experienced clinicians use this phrase for the education of young practitioners, who often go to the most exotic diagnosis first. When determining the cause for an illness, one must consider common pathology (horses) before rare conditions (zebras). I'm going to twist the saying for our purposes.

In the diet world, don't chase after zebras when there is an elephant in the room.

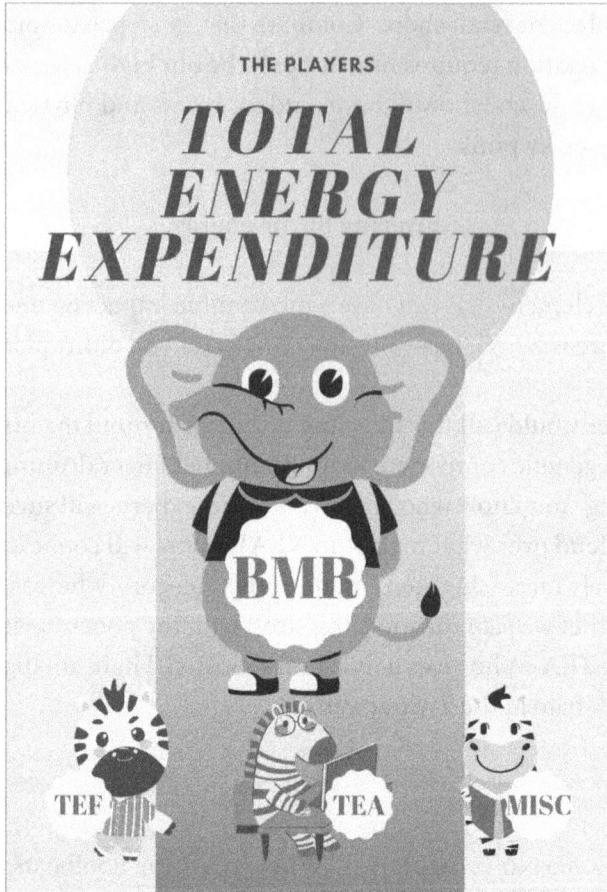

THE PLAYERS

TOTAL ENERGY EXPENDITURE

BMR

TEF   TEA   MISC

Our elephant? BMR. For total Calories used throughout the day,
BMR is the largest energy bucket. Sure, you can increase your TEA.
Maybe you successfully add more NEAT. Fantastic. Movement is
good. Just don't chase after the zebras and forget about our elephant.

～

I've laid out an example for the non-athlete. It helps to visualize the numbers among the acronym vomit. These are *guesstimates* for the average human. If you are Michael Phelps, these are not your values. Is Serena Williams reading? Move along, por favor. Oh, and congrats on your record-breaking U.S. Open wins.

Total Energy Expenditure
75% ~ BMR
10% ~ TEF
10% ~ TEA
5% ~ MISC

100% ~ Maths

Where does that leave us? You cannot change your age or biological sex. Mom and dad determined your predisposition to fidgeting, and I don't recommend a career change to stimulate more shivering.

The answer—walk more, increase skeletal muscle mass, and oh, control your consumption of Calories.

---

1. Moniz, Sara C, et al. "Mechanistic and methodological perspectives on the impact of intense interval training on post-exercise metabolism." *Scand J Med Sci Sports.* 2020 Apr 30 (4): 638-51.

5

TRACKING—FOLLOW THE NUMBERS

Scientists originally developed the hottest chili pepper in the world, Dragon's Breath, for use as an anesthetic to numb the skin.

D id you know that Doritos were originally "trash" from a restaurant in Disneyland? Restaurants used to throw away leftover tortillas. Bothered by this waste, a traveling salesman suggested frying them up and making them into chips. Cooks added a dash of salt, and some special spices. The result—a new hit among the park's visitors. A marketing executive from the food giant, Fritos, discovered this tasty snack, while on a family vacation. He immediately envisioned a prepackaged item that fit nicely in the company's product line. The rest, they say, is history.

The serving size listed on the bag of Cool Ranch Doritos is 28g which is about 12 chips. I'm speculating here, but I highly doubt they became a 5-billion-dollar-a-year consumable with everybody limiting themselves to just eating a handful.

That's the funny thing about "serving size." It's *suggested* and *served* to you, without your input on the matter.

Contrast that with "portion size," which is what you *put* on your *plate*. Portion size is often larger than serving size. When the opposite is true, there is usually a small child and green stuff involved.

Until the 1960s most food was prepared at home. Nutrition information was hard to find and only used for Americans with specific dietary needs. Over the years, the availability of processed foods and bogus marketing claims increased dramatically. As a result, the Food and Drug Administration (FDA) completed a set of consumer guidelines for voluntary nutrition labeling in 1973. The original labels look different from those we see today. I will not use this space to narrate the riveting tale, but I will point out that consumers and their demand for knowledge were the heroes in the story responsible for the evolution of what we see on the box.

~

Decoding Nutrition Labels

In the land of magical fairies and bottomless wine, food labels help you make informed food choices. In reality, they provide you with the information to track what you are consuming.

The FDA requires labels on most packaged foods and beverages. Thankfully, they have a uniform appearance. At the top of the label, you will find the suggested serving size and the total number of servings in the container. They list total Calories in the largest font size. We find macronutrients (fat, carbohydrates, and protein) next. Micronutrients are toward the bottom. For inquiring minds, the list of ingredients (in descending order by weight) floats around somewhere outside the official nutrition box.

The following are my simple rules when reading food labels for tracking:

RULE #1: Determine your serving size.

This is not a guessing game. Do not eye ball or guesstimate. Here, accuracy is required.

RULE #2: Record TOTAL grams of macronutrients.

Don't forget to multiply by number of servings. As for carbs, get out of here with that "net" stuff.

RULE #3: Ignore the % Daily Value.

I don't care that it's in bold. These are not your numbers. They belong to Bob, in accounting at the FDA, who was a guinea pig one fateful day. Not really, but you likely won't have the same macro breakdown as the average fictitious person.

RULE #4: Track everything. And I mean everything.

I once put on an extra pound in a month, because I was not keeping track of my gummy vitamins and chewy supplements. Yes, I sometimes eat like a child. Those Omega-3 bears are delicious, high in Calories, and now banned from my house.

RULE #5: Work with what you have.

For the sake of completeness, I'm sad to inform you that the FDA allows up to 20% variability on reporting. Yep. Labels are not entirely accurate. For example, a serving of food clocking in at 300 Calories could range anywhere from 240 to 360. There is even more of a discrepancy at restaurants. Shockingly, no one is in the back weighing your meal. Since these dinners are usually higher in Calories, it's a double whammy. Don't get discouraged. We have to start somewhere and work with what we have.

Weighing and Logging Food

Have you ever heard the expression, "You are what you eat?" My grandmother used to say that almost every time we sat down to dinner at her house. It usually was in response to me scrunching up my nose as she placed a heaping mound of lima beans on my plate. It didn't matter how much butter she used, I never appreciated the flavor of the little starchy bean.

You are what you eat. Over, and over, and over again. As a small child who still viewed things through a literal filter, I couldn't help but think the last thing in the world I wanted to resemble is a vegetable. As a parent now, I appreciate the sentiment and the meaning behind the expression. I tried using it on my crotch goblins one day, pleading with them to consume a higher amount of green stuff. My youngest quickly explained, "Mommy, if you are what you eat, then I want to be a unicorn cupcake."

A more appropriate expression would be something like, *you are how much you eat.* In modern society, the only way to appreciate what we are consuming is to determine the WHAT and the HOW MUCH.

The WHAT refers to the composition of the food (in terms of fat, protein, and carbohydrates). The HOW MUCH refers to the weight of the food, determined by its portion size.

Now is the time to introduce you to my good buddy, Mr. Food Scale. Ladies, he's a catch—precise with attention to detail, uncomplicated with only a minimal amount of "buttons" to push. A whiz in the kitchen, he barely takes up any counter space. Best of all, he won't let you down like Mr. Serving Cups. Go buy one and make sure you have batteries. It doesn't do you any good to bring him home after your shopping date and not be able to "get him going." Yes, I'm sexualizing kitchen objects. This stuff is super boring to write about, and I'm trying to make it easier to remember.

Let's start with some simple rules and tips. I'll also throw in some more homework for funsies.

RULE #1: Measure by weight, not by volume.

Also known as, my heaping tablespoon is not the same weight as your heaping tablespoon. Plus, it's nowhere near the serving size listed on the food label.

Homework time: Measuring Dry Ingredients
1) Find a dry ingredient in your pantry that has a serving size in both measuring cups and grams. I used 5-minute Quick Grits. Withhold your judgement, Judgy-McJudgerson. On most days, I don't have time or the inclination for the real thing.
2) Set your scale to "grams" and use the "zero" or "tare" button.
3) Weigh the container.
4) Use measuring cups to scoop out a level portion.
5) Reweigh the container and determine the grams of food removed. I can almost guarantee it will not match the grams in the recommended serving size on the container.
6) Conversely, keep the container on the scale and use the measuring cup to remove the grams in one serving. Often, it will not match or fill what you think is a level scoop.

Extra Credit: Measuring Nut Butters
1) Find a wet ingredient in your pantry that has a serving size in both measuring spoons and grams. I used Nutella.
2) Scoop out what you *want* as a serving.
3) Place the rest of the container on the scale to determine its weight.
4) While the container is still on the scale, use a second spoon to remove the exact amount in a recommended serving. It may take you a few tries to match the numbers.

5) Compare the two spoons.

6) Optional: Cry a little inside at the difference.

RULE #2: Weigh food in grams.

There are two major reasons for this requirement. First, as you probably noted from the above challenges, nutrition labels list serving sizes in both volume and weight (usually in grams). I'm not sure about everyone else reading this, but mama doesn't have the time to mess around with converting ounces and grams. Second, it's easier to determine the number of servings if we are using the metric system and dividing by base 10. I have enough fraction fun as a parent of elementary school children. As a result, I'm going to limit its existence in my kitchen as much as possible.

RULE #3: Be consistent.

I have seen entire blog posts and strangers arguing over the interwebs on the best way to use a kitchen scale. I like to weigh meat and protein sources after cooking, since the weight usually decreases as water evaporates and fat cooks out. Grains, rice, and pastas expand during the cooking process because of water absorption; therefore, I like to weigh them dry. Also, the values on most food labels correspond to the dry state of the ingredient. They don't always provide the numbers for the cooked version. Ultimately, you do you boo. Just do it the same way every time.

RULE #4: Weigh the Secret Sauces

It may seem like overkill, but it is very important that you include oils, dressings, and condiments in your tracking. These are some of the most energy-dense (translation: high in Calories) foods you will consume. If you have never paid attention to both the serving size and Calories in these items, you are in for a bit of a shock.

During my first tracking rodeo, I was on a mission to find secret sauces that were both tasty and reasonably low-ish in Calories. I connected with individuals who had undertaken the same quest and picked their brains for their favorite condiments. When cooking at home, I learned many ways to swap ingredients that had similar flavor but better numbers.

Alas, there were some items that had no substitute. I'm looking at you, blue cheese dressing. In those cases, *I either limited my portion or consumed them without guilt.* There is plenty of room on the spectrum between eating a dry salad like a sociopath and using ½ cup of ranch to disguise the taste of veggies like a toddler.

what you record.	what you eat.
PERCEPTION	REALITY
coffee=5 Cal	"coffee"=340 Cal
banana=87 Cal	"banana"=130 Cal
1 serving=120 Cal	"1 serving"=1260 Cal

Homework time: Make a list of your favorite sauces and low-Calorie alternatives.

Finally, I'll leave you with some tips for quickly weighing condiments and meal prepping. Preparing food in advance is a quick and easy way to keep meals available for when you are too hungry to make sound decisions.

TIP: Tracking Oils, Dressings, and Condiments
1) Weigh the entire bottle.
2) Use your desired amount.
3) Zero out the scale.
4) Reweigh the entire bottle and subtract from the original weight.

TIP: Dividing a Large Recipe
1) Zero out a large container.
2) Find the total weight of the finished recipe.
3) Add the ingredients into your food-logging app to calculate macros and Calories.
4) Divide recipe into serving containers.
5) Label each container with total Cal/protein/fat/carbs.

TIP: Meal Prepping for the Week
1) Cook your proteins, starches/grains and veggies separately.
2) Zero out an individual serving container.
3) Add a portion of the cooked protein and record grams.
4) Zero out again.
5) Add a portion of the cooked starch/grains and record grams.
6) Zero out one last time.
7) Add a portion of the vegetables and record grams.
8) Repeat for remaining containers.
9) Label each container with total Cal/protein/fat/carbs.

One of the most common questions in weight loss or training forums is "Why am I not losing weight?" The original poster will often list their daily Calories <insert tiny amount here>, their exercise routine, and how long they've been operating at these numbers. In the most recent example that comes to mind, a young lady was eating 1,200 Cal and exercising approximately 6 hours a week. Before we requested any additional information, some more experienced forum members solved her problem. The answer—she wasn't eating 1,200 Calories. Some more obvious culprits were the many servings of peanut butter (not weighed) and scoops of protein powder in her shakes. Spoiler Alert: The scoop in the tub is a lie!

∿

Tracking food may seem overwhelming at first, but most individuals quickly adapt to a routine. Prepping, weighing, and recording meals or snacks will help you stick with your meal plan for the day. Knowing the Calories in some of your favorite foods may inspire you to practice some creativity and seek other alternatives. Changing your portion size may compel you to appreciate and savor the small bites of your favorite treats. Even if your eating behaviors remain the same, you now have the knowledge of what is going into your body.

Keep in mind that tracking food doesn't have to be a permanent lifestyle change. I only track consistently during periods where I want to reduce scale weight, which only amounts to a few months out of a calendar year.

Stepping on the Scale

The one thing I love about small gyms is the camaraderie that can develop between patrons. Even if you don't know everyone's name, you recognize the 6:00 PM weekday regulars, the early risers, or the mid-shift retirees. It doesn't take much more than a tip of the chin or a brief wave between members for a place to feel like home. Historically, I have been a weeknight warrior, taking a change of clothes every morning and driving straight from work for my evening session. One particular night, I ran into another regular, who I hadn't seen in a while. It was upon my attempt at awkward small talk in the locker room, that she revealed her most recent weight loss.

"I'm so excited! I started this new diet, and I've lost 12 pounds in 4 days," she exclaimed.

"Most of that is water weight," the demon on my shoulder whispered. "She'll gain it all back and then some as soon as she falls off the low-carb wagon."

The sad truth of the matter is that she regained the "weight" back and lost the motivation to continue on with the plan. How many of you have been in similar situations? Have ridden the roller coaster highs and lows of the scale? "Did everything right" only for the scale to go up the next time you check?

Before we dig into the more common reasons for scale fluctuations, we need to address body composition. The human body is sub-divided into fat mass and fat-free mass. This isn't rocket science. Fat mass is, well, fat. That leaves fat-free mass as everything else. This includes muscle, bone, connective tissue (ligaments and tendons connecting muscle to bone), organs, WATER, and anything in your digestive tract. If we are splitting hairs, this differs slightly from lean body mass (LBM), which includes the small amount of essential fat in organs and bone marrow.

I don't care how many hours a day you lift weights, your body is not adding pounds of muscle overnight. Education is important, but it won't double your brain volume. And calcium supplements won't lead you to change your Facebook status to "big-boned." Therefore, most of the *daily* fluctuations you experience on the scale result from changes in water weight and whatever is in your digestive system.

In a sad, ironic twist, the food and liquid you consume weighs some-thing. Finish the water in your super special monogrammed tumbler? Add 2 lbs to the scale. That cheesecake you had for dessert has the equivalent weight of a brick. I'm not advocating anyone switch to a diet of toast, air, and lettuce.

Remember, what you put in your body shows up on the scale.

On the flip side, the numbers reflect what comes out of your body, too. The daily sacrifice to the porcelain gods, the 4 lbs of sweat you lost in your high-intensity dance cycle hot yoga boot camp class, even the loogie you hocked on your trail run all decrease your daily readings.

Water retention affects scale weight.

Did you meet some friends for Friday night appetizers (high in salt and carbohydrates) plus adult beverages? Cue Saturday morning bloat. Stressed out? One of the many actions of cortisol, the alarm hormone, is to increase water weight. Did your doctor prescribe a new medication? That softness in your ankles could be a side effect. Too little sleep? Not only are you going to want to binge all day, but also the lack of shut eye affects your kidneys, which regulate salt and water balance. For all my menstruating ladies out there, normal vari-ations in hormones during your cycle affect water weight. A rule of thumb, your body keeps more water when it is preparing to drop an egg (ovulation) or cast off your oven's lining (menstruation).

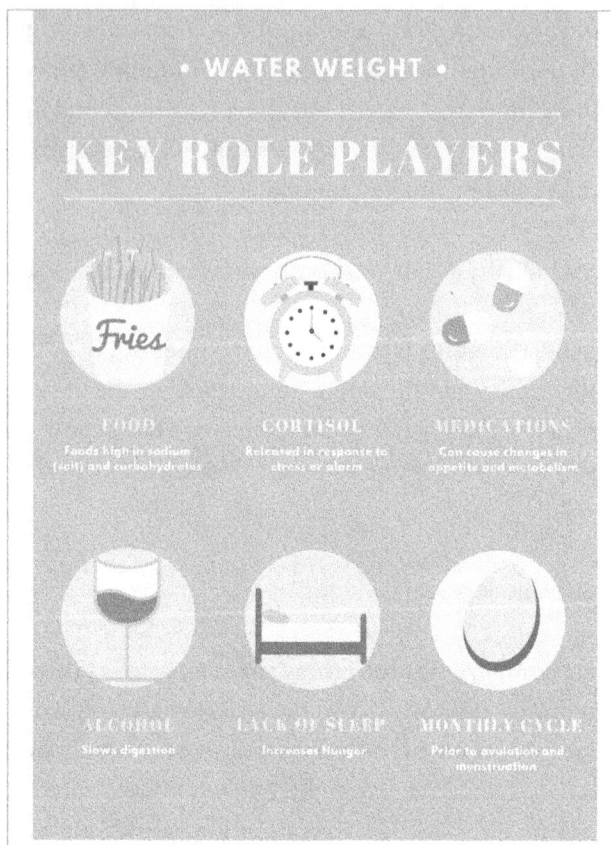

• WATER WEIGHT •

KEY ROLE PLAYERS

FOOD
Foods high in sodium (salt) and carbohydrates

CORTISOL
Released in response to stress or alarm

MEDICATIONS
Can cause changes in appetite and metabolism

ALCOHOL
Slows digestion

LACK OF SLEEP
Increases Hunger

MONTHLY CYCLE
Prior to ovulation and menstruation

Even with all the daily fluctuations, it is worthwhile to track your scale weight. Here's how it's done:

Use the same scale (on a hard surface), on the same day of the week, at a similar time, while wearing minimal clothing (or none).

I'm a morning coffee drinker, so I prefer to step on the scale after my second cup. Yes, dear reader, I opt for a psychological win via my pooping schedule.

You can either track daily or pick 2 days of the week to weigh yourself.

For the twice-a-week approach, I recommend Wednesdays and Sundays. Once you've collected your data, you can either average the numbers or leave them alone. Either way, resist the urge to detect a trend until you collect at least 3 weeks' worth of measurements.

I'll leave you with one final disclaimer. For individuals with eating disorders or disordered habits, ditch the scale. If the thought of weighing yourself causes anxiety, either skip this item entirely or have a trusted family member/friend do it for you. A simple tool should never be the source of stress and unhealthy behaviors.

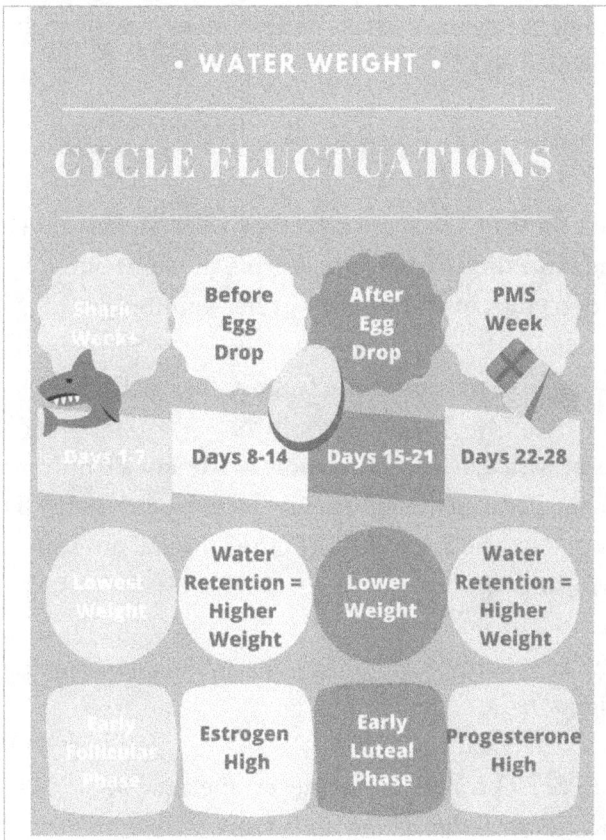

• WATER WEIGHT •

CYCLE FLUCTUATIONS

Shark Weeks	Before Egg Drop	After Egg Drop	PMS Week
Days 1-7	Days 8-14	Days 15-21	Days 22-28
Lowest Weight	Water Retention = Higher Weight	Lower Weight	Water Retention = Higher Weight
Early Follicular Phase	Estrogen High	Early Luteal Phase	Progesterone High

Taking Body Measurements and Progress Photos
Once a month, I recommend taking body measurements and
progress photos. Over a long period, the goal is to have a linear
decrease in weight. For many, this will not be a perfectly straight line.
Don't become discouraged, focusing only on the scale. The numbers,
by themselves, may not paint an accurate picture.

Body measurements and progress photos will tell the actual story.
Sometimes, the scale weight may stay the same (or have a minimal
decrease) but there are inches lost all over the body. I love seeing the
progress photos of folks standing in their old pair of pants. If you lost
3 pant sizes or fit into an old favorite shirt, does it really matter what
how much you weigh?

Take photos and measurements every 4 weeks.

I like to take mine on the same day of the week, in the same location,
around the same time of day, and wearing the same outfit. Relax your
body and don't tuck in your tummy or flex your biceps.

Take photos of the front, side, and back.

This is easier with a helper, but a selfie in front of a bathroom mirror
will work, too. For measurements, use a soft tape measure. These are
only a few dollars and are well worth the minimal investment. Record
the following areas:

1) CHEST: Measure around the widest part, usually at the
headlights, ladies.

2) BICEPS: Pick a side (overachievers measure both). Measure
halfway between the armpit and elbow.

3) WAIST: Wrap the tape measure around the tummy about 1
inch above the belly button.

4) HIPS: With your heels together, wrap the tape measure around the largest part of your booty.

5) THIGHS: Wrap the tape measure around the widest part. Again, overachievers may measure both.

Remember, photos and measurements will reveal progress over longer periods of time. On the flip side, it will not have the same roller coaster-like readings and associated anxiety as stepping on that little slab of plastic in your bathroom. Just keep reminding yourself that you didn't put the weight on in 30 days; therefore, expecting everything to melt off in a month is just insanity.

Journaling for Post-Teen Years

What is your relationship with food? Does it consume your thoughts? Do you use it as a reward and treat yo' self? Does negative self talk come out every time you eat?

Food surrounds us. With so many quick, delicious options, it's easy to become divorced from eating to survive. That's why I recommend taking a moment to define your relationship with food. Is it a healthy one? How much brain space does eating occupy? Are they negative thoughts or positive ones?

Your next homework assignment is to keep a *written* journal of what I refer to as *The Whys of Eating*. It's a chance to explore your relationship with food and uncover the emotions linked to your eating habits.

Keep a hand-written log of your eating habits for 30 days.

Write WHAT you eat. Include the food, macronutrient breakdown, and Calories. It seems redundant to write this information down when you've already logged it in an app. However, it's nice to refer back to what you ate and link it with your feelings. Did you feel full eating that new chicken marsala recipe? Did it leave you feeling tired, drowsy, and wanting a nappy nap? It's easier to connect those sensations with a tangible meal as opposed to just an entry that says "dinner."

WHEN did you eat your meal or snack? Did you follow a pattern all week or did your eating habits change daily? Are you in the habit of eating late at night? Do you reach for a snack an hour after lunch? What are your trends? Pay attention to any bad habits that emerge. Maybe you waited too long between meals and then gorged on late lunches. Does eating earlier or later correlate with fluctuations in energy levels? Include times in your food journal and then look at the data to see if there is anything you might change.

The next step is to log WHERE you eat. Do you eat most of your meals at the kitchen table or on the couch? Sit in a chair or lie down in bed? I eat while I cook. There are a lot of "pregame" Calories when I taste-test our meals. I'm notorious for nibbling so much while in the kitchen I'm rarely hungry by the time I sit down with the family. Notice any trends? How many Calories do you consume while chilling on the couch versus sitting at the dining room table? You can break many bad habits by moving to a different location.

Now, write WHY you ate. This step is the hardest and will force you to examine your relationship with food. Be honest and thorough. I don't want to see "dinner time." Even if it is a scheduled meal with the family, write what it means to you. "I'm hungry, and I'm able to enjoy this meal with my loved ones," conveys more information and meaning than "routine supper."

Do you eat when stressed? Note in your journal that your snack is for comfort, not fuel. Are there large chunks of time when you are skipping meals? I've encountered many friends and coworkers who eat less when they are under pressure. Watch out for this habit as it may lead to overeating when you do finally take a break. What about treating yo' self? This is big for me. Payday? Bam—you get some ice cream. Knocked your work presentation out of the park? Bam—girl, go dig out that hidden chocolate in the back of the freezer. Personally, I don't have a problem with treats, but if you are reaching for sugar every time you put on pants or pay a bill, it might be time to reexamine the habit.

On a more serious note, this is just an exercise to dig a little deeper into your relationship with food. If you find trends associated with frequent negative emotions, please reach out to your healthcare provider, as it might be time to work with a professional to find positive ways to work through these difficult emotions.

Finally, *RATE* your hunger when finished. Instead of "full" or "still hungry" or "stuffed," use a percentage. Did you put your fork down at 80% full or were you at critical capacity? Are you leaving the table satisfied? What is your personal comfort level with "fullness" at the end of the meal? Can you go about your life at 60-70% fullness or do you *need* to rub your food belly before you stand up?

I have a terrible habit of wolfing down my portions. It takes a minute for the comfortable feeling of fullness to register in my brain. I'm shoveling things too quickly for my feedback loop to be effective. I've learned that I really need to stop eating when I'm about 50-60% full. Yes, I eat that quickly. No, I don't always chew. It's allowed me to develop an immunity to brain freeze.

For the sake of completeness, I recommend checking back 20 minutes after you finish the meal. Are you still stuffed? Is it still uncomfortable to move? Or do you feel satisfied?

FOOD JOURNAL

WHAT	Item and Quantity
WHEN	Time of Day
WHERE	Location and Position
WHY	Hungry, Reward, Stress...
% FULL	Immediately After & 20 Min Later

30 DAY CHALLENGE

That's it for the food part of your journal. Here are 5 additional entries to include:

1) Commit to moving.
Are you meeting a friend for spin class one morning? Great. Schedule it. Are you trying a new rock-climbing gym? Fantastic. Write it down. Are you riding bikes around the neighborhood with your kiddos? Fabulous. Put it in your notebook. Stop relying on motivation to exercise. Plan it!

2) Record your step count, including targets.
How much are you walking? This is one of the easiest targets to change. Find out what you are averaging now and add 2,000 more

steps. Once you've consistently hit the higher goal, add another 2,000. This is an excellent case of "more is more."

3) Track your entire menstrual cycle, not just shark week.
Where are you in your cycle? Before egg drop? After shark week? You need not list the specific day, but it's important to have a rough idea where you are and what you should be expecting. This will allow you to link changes in scale weight to specific times in your cycle. Do your eating habits change depending on the phase? It may not prevent you from stuffing your face with greasy foods, but at least you will understand the cause of the cravings.

4) Let go of your worries.
Twice a week make space to acknowledge your worries. Pick the days in advance and label an area in your journal or notebook for you to jot down your thoughts. Writing provides an opportunity to organize overwhelming feelings. Negative emotions pour out on paper and give you a chance to analyze the situation in a more logical manner.

5) Find five positive things.
This is not a "gratitude" entry. They don't have to be profound. Yes, I know you are grateful for your family, friends, and good health. But pay attention to the tiny, upbeat incidents that happen every day. Did you wear a favorite pair of earrings? Were you happy to beat the rain into work? Did you finish that last load of laundry? Maybe your child brushed his teeth without a reminder. Positive thinking breeds positive thinking. Recognize and focus on these joyous occasions.

~

Undoubtedly, this is a lot of information to record. Think of journaling as another tool in your tool belt. Try it for 30 days, longer if you desire. It's not a practice that you need to continue indefinitely. Pick what items you wish to maintain beyond the first month. For instance, I haven't stopped scheduling my workouts at the beginning of the week. It has kept me accountable, even when motivation is low. Find what works for you and make it a habit.

Jumping off the Tracking Train

Calorie counting, macronutrient tracking, and journaling will become less burdensome with time. Create shortcuts. Save favorite foods. Make documenting reflexive. These will all eventually become habits in your daily routine.

But should they be permanent? Are these changes something you will continue even after you've achieved your desired weight loss? Personally, I do not track my intake unless I have a specific reason. When I have an upcoming competition or my work pants are fitting too snugly, I dust off the kitchen scale and determine my new starting measurements. Between these times, I use the following tips and tricks.

Include protein with every meal or snack.

To reach my targets when I am tracking, I almost always need to eat protein with every snack or meal. Aim for 4 or more servings a day. For meats, I recommend using your palm for rough estimates.

Consume at least 5 servings of vegetables a day.

Here, I consider a serving size to equal your fist. For salads or leafy greens, one serving is 2 fists.

Add 2 fruits or 2 grains.

I try not to complicate the serving size on this. You can use the entire actual fruit as one serving (i.e. a banana). For small fruits or grains, you can estimate with a fist. Dried fruit is the exception. Use about ½ the size of an open palm. Remember, water plays a role in energy density, and the dehydration process removes most of it. This leaves the same number of Calories in a smaller package. If you prefer a higher carb intake (either for training or preference), bump this up to 3-4 servings a day.

Eat a meal in four "courses."

You don't have to prepare 4 separate courses. Dirtying extra dishes is silly. Just eat your meal in order of importance. Veggies are first, followed by meat or protein source. If you are still hungry, fill up on your grains. I have a sweet tooth, so fruit at the end of the meal satisfies my cravings.

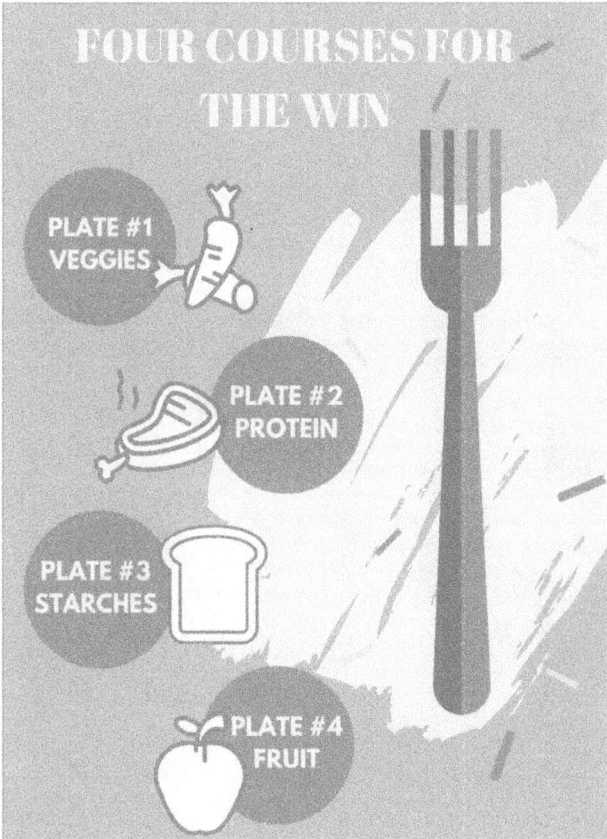

FOUR COURSES FOR THE WIN

PLATE #1 VEGGIES

PLATE #2 PROTEIN

PLATE #3 STARCHES

PLATE #4 FRUIT

6

THE NUMBERS DON'T LIE—
DETERMINING CALORIE REQUIREMENTS

Graham crackers were invented to quell sexual urges.

The average beaver dam is 5 feet tall and 330 feet wide. Like your mama. Sorry, couldn't resist. Personally, I find beavers to be fascinating creatures that are cute and cuddly. Mother Nature, however, has deemed them chubby and ungraceful on land. A prey animal for wolves, bears, etc., these resourceful engineers manipulate their environment for protection and to secure easy access to food during winter months. They use their iron-infused front teeth to chop down large trees near rivers and streams. The resultant blockage creates a pond, or still body of water, where aquatic plants thrive, and in colder months, the deeper water allows beavers to dive under the ice layer for their sustenance.

In the thick wilderness of northern Alberta, the largest dam ever built is 2,790 feet long. We even see it from space. Like your mama. Really, these jokes write themselves. Typically, beavers stay in the same location until their food supply diminishes. Next to the dam, they build their home, or beaver lodge, in the waterway's bank. These dome-shaped structures house a single, monogamous couple, their offspring, and their offspring from the previous season. Imagine the size of the metropolis supported by a configuration of vegetation more than twice the length of the Hoover Dam.

Beavers are the modern decedents of ROUSs. From the movie, *The Princess Bride*, Rodents of Unusual Size are one of the three major hazards in the Fire Swamp. If you haven't already, do yourself a favor and watch one of the best movies of all time. *Castoroides*, rodents from the Ice age, grew up to 8 feet long and weighed in around 200 pounds. They were plus-sized prey for plus-sized predators, like the saber-tooth tiger. Similar to beavers of today, they were herbivores and had large incisors (up to 6 inches) used for gnawing. Ecological changes, along with the hunting practices of early North American settlers, hastened their extinction.

Food and perfume manufacturers have been using castoreum as an additive for at least 90 years. Castoreum is a chemical compound stored in the beaver's castor sacs, which are between the pelvis and the base of the tail. Do you know what else is between the pelvis and tail base? Ding, ding, ding. You got it! Castoreum is beaver butt goo. You'd think a combination of castor gland secretions, anal gland secretions, and urine would have an unpleasant funk. Nope. Because of a beaver's unique diet of leaves and bark, their brown booty slime has a vanilla scent, which is why scientists incorporate it into their recipes. This lends an entirely different spin to the phrase, "natural flavoring."

~

Choosing Weekly Fat Loss Goals
As much as I would love to continue our slightly inappropriate side quest about beavers, it's time to learn how to calculate daily and weekly Calorie goals.

Continuing along with our Calories IN = Calories OUT model, to lose mass, one must be in a *caloric deficit*. The opposite is also true. One needs a Calorie surplus to increase mass.

The body requires a Calorie deficit to lose mass.

Notice, I did not say weight. Do not confuse scale weight with true loss of body mass. Equally important, I did not say fat. While the aim is to lose fat mass, we expect a small amount of skeletal muscle loss. An even sadder truth, individuals can lose mass (including changes in scale weight and appearance) but still have the same body fat percentage. Don't believe me? Here is our first math example:

John starts his weight loss journey at 200 lbs total with fat contributing 40 lbs.
John is at 20% body fat.
John loses 35 lbs of mass.
Go, John!
Of those 35 lbs lost, 7 lbs are fat.
At 165 lbs (with 33 lbs of fat remaining), John is still at 20% body fat.
John is now *skinny fat*. I don't particularly care for this term, but it is very descriptive.
Don't be like John.

Obviously, these are hypothetical numbers used to fit a narrative, but the example illustrates the point that weight loss is not always equal to fat loss. So how do we determine a Calorie deficit in the first place? Fortunately for all of us, science has already done The Maths. Drum roll, please.

We require a 3,500 Calorie deficit to lose a pound of fat.

The 3,500 Calorie Rule is conventional weight-loss wisdom. Scientists wrote about it over 6 decades ago. It's a simple rule of thumb from which we will base all of our calculations.

Since there are 7 days in a week, a daily deficit of 500 Calories will cause 1 lb of weight loss a week or 52 lbs in a year. For those in the back of the class, 3,500 Calories/7 days = 500 Calories.

A simple way to set Calorie targets is to determine the daily or weekly deficits required to reach your goals.

TARGET #1: We need a daily deficit of 250 Cal to lose 0.5 lb a week.

OR

TARGET #2: We need a daily deficit of 500 Cal to lose 1 lb a week.

OR

TARGET #3: We need a daily deficit of 1000 Cal to lose 2 lbs a week.

Over the course of 1 year, a person could lose 26 lbs, 52 lbs, or 104 lbs, respectively. These are all very admirable targets. However, the ability to achieve any of these goals depends on perseverance. Or how well you embrace the suck.

Can you see where I'm leading you? Step one is simply to determine your overall weight loss goal and the time you wish to accomplish it. Do you want to lose 0.5, 1, or 2 pounds a week? Are you getting ready for a family vacation in a month and want to rock a bikini, or do you have all winter to work toward your summer physique? You now have the information to pick your daily deficit target.

The one thing you are missing, and it's a biggie, is your Maintenance Calorie consumption. When eating at Maintenance Calories, you are neither gaining mass nor losing mass. This is our starting point of all calculations, and the last step is to subtract your daily deficit target from your daily maintenance number, and voilà! You have your daily Calorie goals.

Maintenance - Deficit = Daily Calorie Goal

This brings us to our second math problem of the day. Unlike the hypothetical example with John, these are my personal numbers from when I first started tracking. These are my maintenance numbers, prior to my first kickboxing match. For reference, I was walking around roughly 165 lbs (a tall 5'11") and training fairly heavily. I was far enough out from my bout I didn't need to cut weight quickly. I also wanted to keep my Calories on the higher end (while still in a deficit) so my workouts didn't suffer.

Melissa starts her journey at 2,050 Calorie maintenance.
Melissa eats in a daily deficit of 250 Calories.
Melissa's daily target of 1,800 Calories is bearable.
Melissa doesn't get hangry or snap off the heads of coworkers and family members.
Melissa consistently loses 0.5 lbs a week.
Melissa is happy at first but frustrated she is not losing more.
Melissa refuses to eat at 1,550 Calories daily.
Don't have unrealistic expectations, like Melissa.

This is the disconnect that many of you will face. Everything looks fantastic on paper, but you will learn quickly (usually in the first 10 days) whether the daily deficit target you chose is realistic. I made a choice and picked the easiest one. And if I'm honest, it took an embarrassingly long time to accept that while I wanted to shed the pounds faster, I wasn't willing to sacrifice the tacos. For you, replace taco with any other pleasure. It could be wine, donuts, or glorious hunks of cheese.

Estimating Maintenance Calories

So how do you calculate Maintenance Calories? I keep dancing around this subject, mainly because I don't believe there is a good way to determine yours. Sure, there are formulas. Except for the BMR calculators, they are not very accurate. Why? There is too much variability between individuals. And everyone is over-estimating how much they move throughout the day.

No-Drama Llama:
Throw out the complicated formulas for maintenance Calorie estimation.

This leaves us with the following two choices:

OPTION #1: Just Track

That's it. Just start logging your current Calorie consumption. Be honest and don't change your current eating habits. Really *see* the amount of fuel you are putting into the equation. Start tracking your scale weight. Is some of that energy going into long-term storage? Or are things staying fairly level? The trouble (and downside) to this method is that it takes time and patience. Everyone wants to jump in with both feet and start the *diet*. I get it.

Immediate results are all the rage, but I implore you to give it 3 weeks. 21 days. This gives you time to develop the skill-set of Calorie tracking and to learn the art of taking body measurements. It will prevent you from becoming overwhelmed while learning how to read a nutrition label, how to use a kitchen scale, and how to document your progress.

OPTION #2: Target Ideal Body Weight x 13

For those of you who cannot *live* without some target, use the above formula to start. What do I mean by Ideal Body Weight? While I'm never a fan of using scale weight as a goal, it can be a useful tool for estimation. Do you have a weight that you would just love to reach?

Maybe the last time you saw those numbers was prior to procreation. Perhaps it's the weight that allows you to fit into your favorite sexy pants, which you haven't worn since your club-hoping days. Whatever your rationale, pick a number that your primary care doctor would approve. Then multiply by 13.

Here's the kicker, though. You still have to track. For 3 weeks. 21 days. Gotcha.

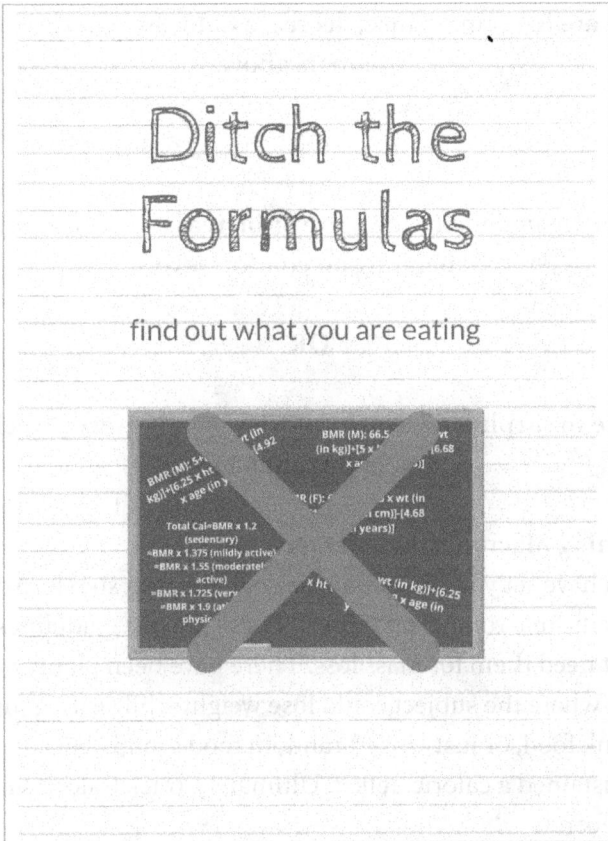

It's decision tree time. Which way are your numbers trending? Are you at maintenance? Did your weight stay the same on the scale, or did it go up or down? If your weight is trending higher, you are most likely in a Calorie surplus. If your weight is trending lower, you are in a Calorie deficit. This is the reason we need 3 weeks worth of tracking. We have to look for trends, not daily snapshots in time.

Uncertain of the direction of weight change after 3 weeks? Go another week. The 3-week recommendation is not a hard-and-fast rule. It's just the bare minimum of time in which to base any decisions. Where do we go from here?

If you are in maintenance, decrease Calories by target deficit numbers above.

OR

If you are in deficit, stay there or increase/decrease targets, depending on comfort levels.

OR

If you are in surplus, decrease Calories by 10% every 3 weeks until you hit maintenance.

Determining Macronutrient Targets

Once you have set your daily Caloric goal, the next step is to determine specific macronutrient targets. These are just guidelines, and we do not need them for mass loss. There have been plenty of instances where the subject could lose weight while eating just meat, or just junk food, or just <insert random food group> because that person sustained a calorie deficit. Ultimately, track Calories first and macros second.

Macronutrient Calorie Conventions
1 gram of protein = 4 Calories
1 gram of carbohydrate = 4 Calories
1 gram of fat = 9 Calories
1 gram of alcohol = 7 Calories

Protein is King

With macro divisions, protein is king. This is the first target you should always set. I recommend 1 gram of protein per pound of *ideal* body weight. Let's set up our third hypothetical math problem.

Meet Sara.
Sara is 180 lbs and would love to fit back into her favorite pair of skinny jeans.
Sara figures her ideal weight is 140 lbs.
For Sara, 140 lbs isn't what she was in her 20s, but it's the weight she can move around well and not get exhausted going up steps.
Sara sets her protein target at 140 grams (560 Calories).
Sara has determined that 1,650 is her daily Calorie target.
This puts Sara's intake at ~34% protein.

There are some key points I would like to highlight in the above example. One, 140 grams of protein may seem like a lot, but strategically divided between meals and snacks, it is entirely achievable. Two, focus on the percent protein in this example. A realistic goal is 30-40% of your daily allotment of Calories. And three, the 1 gram per 1 lb of ideal body weight is ideal for keeping muscle mass high. You can go lower or higher, depending on your preferences. Don't want to bother with a calculation. Here is a simple guideline for females:

For Females:
50 grams of protein = minimum (GOOD)
120 grams of protein = middle ground (BETTER)
1 gram protein/1 lb ideal body weight = target (BEST)

The guidelines for males are similar. The major difference is the "middle ground" is a bit higher.

For Males:
50 grams of protein = minimum (GOOD)
150 grams of protein = middle ground (BETTER)
1 gram protein/1 lb ideal body weight = target (BEST)

Fat is the Heir

If protein is king, then fat is next in line to the throne. Recall, both protein and fat are essential macronutrients. Once we nail down protein, it's time to set fat targets.

Target 50 grams of fat daily.

A good range for fat would be anywhere from 45 to 75 grams, with 25-35% of your daily Caloric intake coming from this macronutrient. Remember, fat is energy dense compared to carbohydrates and protein, so use the correct multiplier. Returning to Sara,

Sara likes red meat and fatty fish.
Sara sets her fat target at 60 grams, which is 540 Calories.
Sara remembered to multiply 60 grams by 9.
Go, Sara.
Sara has determined that 1,650 is her daily Calorie target.
This puts Sasha's intake at ~33% fat.

Carbohydrates are Peasants

We allot the remaining Calories for carbohydrates. THE END.

∾

It should be that simple. But... I challenge everyone to experiment with your carbohydrate and fat ratios. Keep protein and total Calories the same.

How do you feel on higher fat, lower carb days? What about higher carb, lower fat? What are your energy levels? Do you feel full? Is it difficult to prepare or choose meals following a particular macronutrient breakdown?

These are all variables that many of us don't pay attention to regularly. It may sound cliché, but *listen to your body*. We will finish Sara's example by assigning the left over Calories all to carbohydrates.

> Sara has targeted 560 Cal for protein and 540 Cal for fat.
> Sara started with 1,650 Calories total.
> This puts Sara's carbohydrate target at 550 Calories (1,650 minus 560 minus 540).
> Sara divides 550 Calories by 4.
> Sara's Calorie target for carbohydrates is 138.

In our example above, our carbohydrate intake is at approximately 33 percent. If you follow the recommendations, the macronutrient pie will end up approximately 1/3 carbs, 1/3 fat and 1/3 protein, which is a very manageable place to be.

Order of Operations
1) Hit Calorie targets first.
2) Knock out daily protein goal, staying within allotted total Calories.
3) Aim for specific fat and carbohydrate targets.

∼

Weekly Cycles
We have only discussed daily targets and deficit goals. However, this view is too myopic for the sake of practicality. Most of us schedule our lives in weekly increments, so our Calorie planning should follow suit.

Once you determine daily targets, multiply by 7 to find the weekly total.

Think of this weekly goal as a pot of Calories that you can divide in any manner that works best with your particular lifestyle.

I've listed some of the most common cycles as examples (complete with cute animal names to aid in memory recall), along with the one major pitfall that is all too prevalent.

～

Slow and Steady Sloth Cycle

This weekly cycle is the easiest to calculate and the one I suggest everyone use in the beginning.

In the example graph, the daily Calorie target is 2,000 (or 14,000 for the entire week).

The Slow and Steady Sloth cycle allots the same number of Calories every day. Stay here for a few weeks and note how it feels.

How is your energy? Hunger levels? Do you need to increase or decrease your Calories for sustainability? Answer these questions first before you start varying your daily numbers.

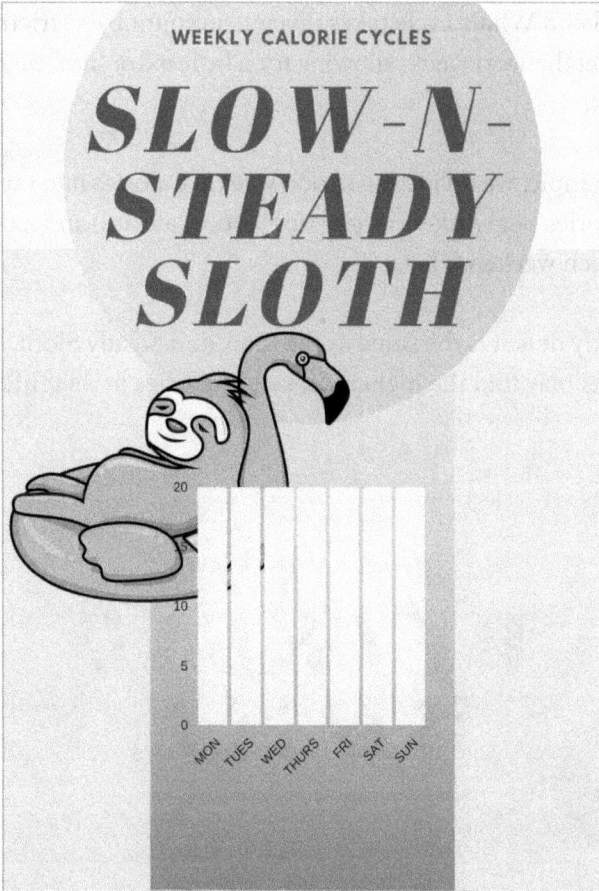

WEEKLY CALORIE CYCLES

SLOW-N-STEADY SLOTH

Weekend Whale

This is a very common cycle that works well for the Monday through Friday, 9 to 5, folks. It's easy following restricted Calories while on a rigid work schedule. Routine alarm clocks, planned meal times, and structured activities lend themselves to greater adherence to lower targets. Once the weekend rolls around along with relaxation, social gatherings, and more free time, the Calories have a habit of increasing.

The Weekend Whale cycle takes this into account by restricting Calories during the workweek, allowing for a little extra "fun" on the weekends.

In our example, we divide the 14,000 weekly Calories into targets of 1,200 Calories per work-week day (for 6,000 Calories) and 4,000 Calories for each weekend day.

The weekly deficit is the same as the Slow and Steady Sloth, but some folks may find the higher weekend Calories fit their lifestyle better.

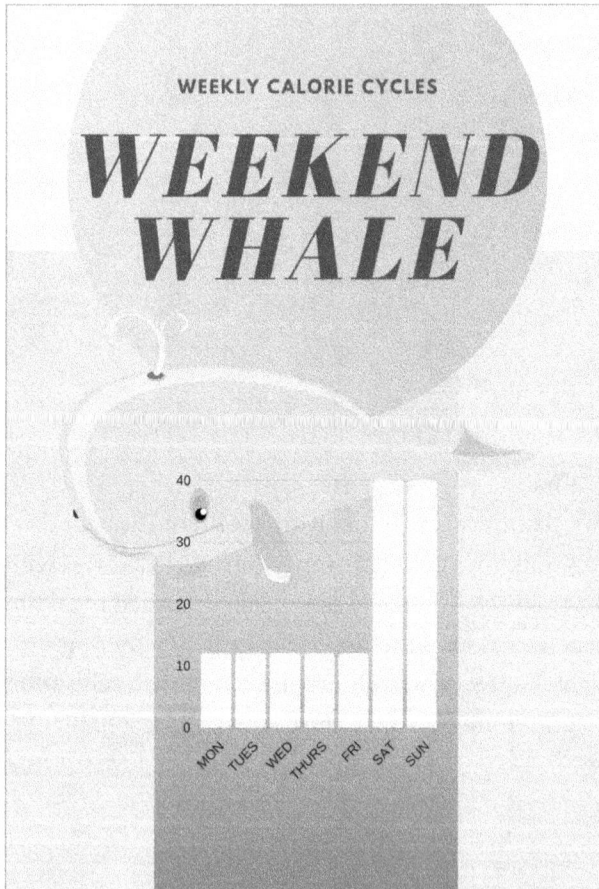

WEEKLY CALORIE CYCLES

WEEKEND WHALE

Party Pig

This is a more extreme allocation of weekly Calories than the Weekend Whale. The Party Pig cycle lends itself nicely for special occasions with rich, celebratory fare, such as birthdays or holidays.

In our example, we restrict the other 6 days of the week to 1,500 Calories (for 9,000 Calories total) with a one-day blow out at 5,000.

The restricted days will be more tolerable than the Weekend Whale. The most difficult aspect of this cycle is just getting right back at the lower deficit and not letting the one day of high Calories inadvertently carry over into multiple days.

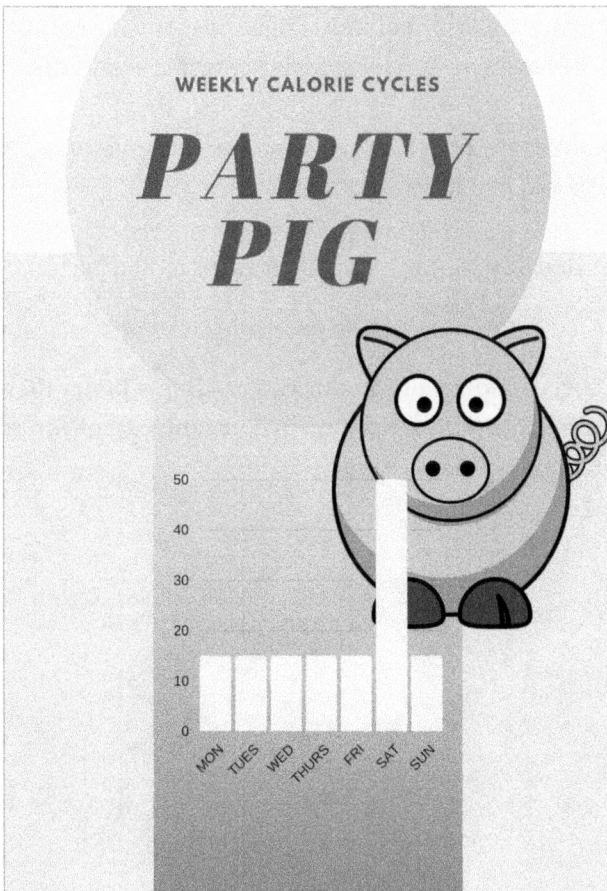

WEEKLY CALORIE CYCLES

PARTY PIG

Yo-Yo Yak
Up and down. Up and down.

Once you have a feel for the Slow and Steady Sloth cycle, the Yo-Yo Yak should be the next challenge.

You will feel fantastic on the higher Calorie days, as the numbers are likely approaching maintenance. The lower days are slightly more tolerable than Party Pig or Weekend Whale because you only have to make it one day before you feel fed again.

This is a fantastic schedule for those who have high training demands. You can allot higher Calories on training days, to assist with hunger and energy demands. Or, I prefer the lower Calories on those days because my hunger signals are worse a day later.

In this example, our high Calorie days have an allotment of 2,375, where the lower days are at 1,500 Calories.

This is just one way we can change our carbs to fit a personal training schedule.

Nutrition social media will call this carb cycling. I prefer the term Calorie cycling, but if we keep protein constant, carbohydrates are the easiest macronutrient to manipulate.

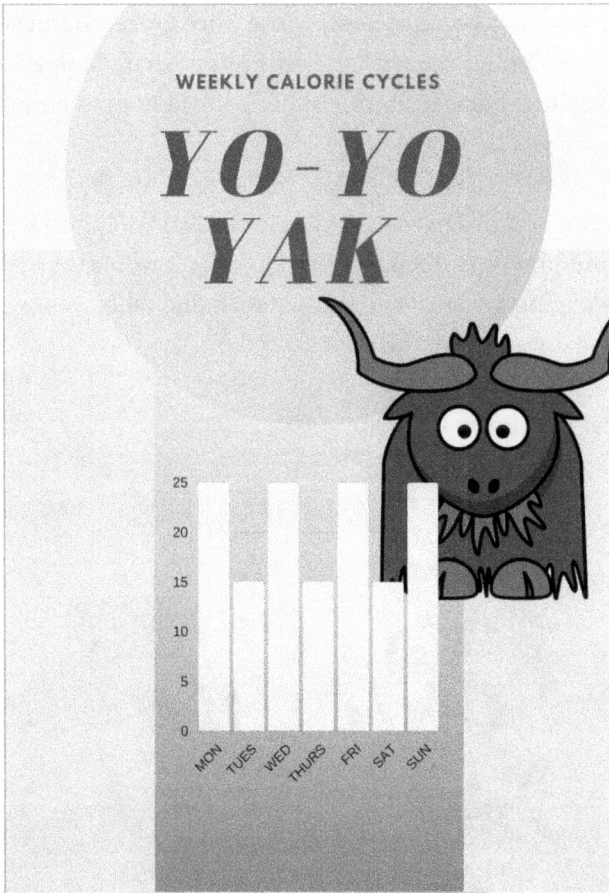

WEEKLY CALORIE CYCLES

YO-YO YAK

Unwitting Unicorn
This is a very common pitfall that many dieters make.

In our scenario, the Unwitting Unicorn did well all week. She adhered to her daily deficit and stuck with her 2,000 Calorie target. Go, girl! Then the weekend hit. She wanted to *reward* herself with some tasty treats for accomplishing her goals. Or she just didn't want to track her weekend consumption. Or our unicorn logged her food but didn't add her adult beverages. You get the gist. Regardless of the reason, she consumed an extra 1,250 Calories a day. Sounds like a lot, right?

One extra-large smoothie at her favorite Juice Queen stand is all it takes one day. Dinner out with the girls plus a shared appetizer puts her over on the other. This brought her back to her maintenance intake for the week.

Miss Unicorn gets discouraged because she was "doing so well" with tracking and planning during the week. What's worse than inadvertently sabotaging her own efforts? Not realizing what went wrong because she doesn't have the data to analyze.

Don't be an Unwitting Unicorn.

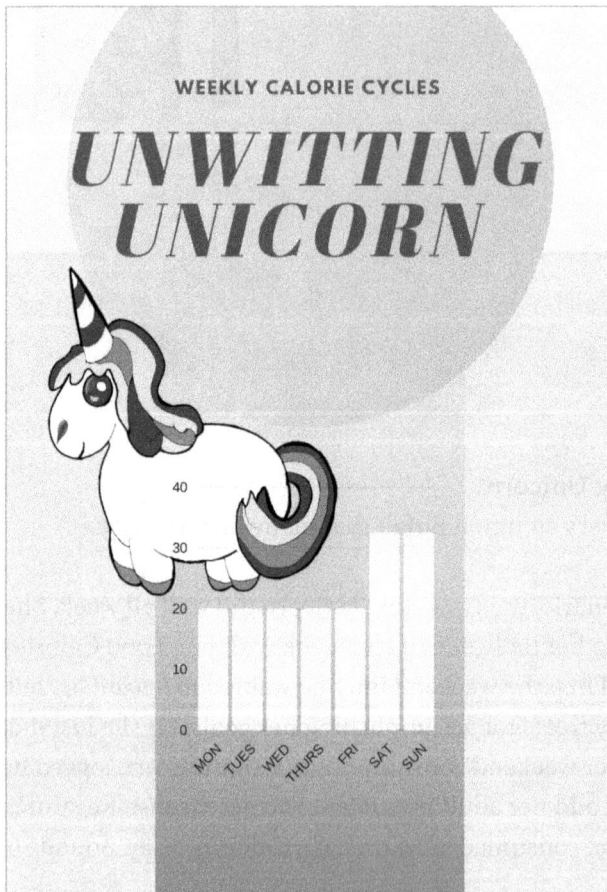

WEEKLY CALORIE CYCLES

UNWITTING UNICORN

~

Myth-Busting Mermaid Takes the Mic
Some of the biggest crocks of dung that pervade pop culture weight
loss media are around meal sizing and meal timing.

Have you ever tried to eat 6 small meals a day? Like a hobbit. It is
possible to feel as if you are eating all the time, but never satisfied or
full.

What about the opposite? Fasting and feasting. It's a swinging
pendulum between insane hunger and food-baby uncomfortable.
Let's just feel miserable all the time.

Myth-Busting Mermaid:
Many small meals are not superior to several large ones.[1, 2, 3]

Are you starving when you first wake up or prefer not to eat until
your first break of the day? If you want to put cash in your wallet
several times a day, perfect.

Prefer to wait until later in the day to run to the bank? Do it.

Get paid in one sizeable sum upon completion of a project?
Outstanding. Toss those Benjamins in the bank account.

Myth-Busting Mermaid:
Thermodynamics doesn't care about how often you eat.[4, 5]

I'll round it out with one last math example.

Meet Marcus.
Marcus has calculated his daily target to be 2,100 Calories.
Marcus's friend tells him to *keep his metabolism up* by eating 6
small meals of 350 Calories each.

This is the *only thing* that worked for his friend.
Marcus works a 12-hour shift without a gazillion breaks.
Marcus ignores his friend.
Marcus eats 3 larger meals of 700 Calories each.
Marcus loses weight.
Be like Marcus.

In our example, 2,100 Calories is 2,100 Calories. Thermodynamics doesn't care how often you put energy in the system or how you divide your fuel. We are all special snowflakes, with special schedules, and special preferences. Find a strategy that works best for your lifestyle.

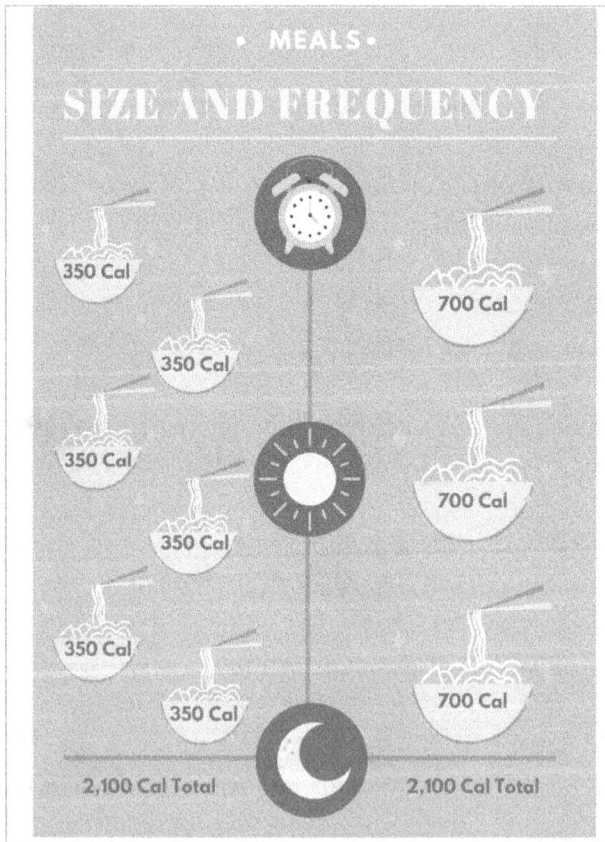

• MEALS •

SIZE AND FREQUENCY

350 Cal
700 Cal
350 Cal
350 Cal
700 Cal
350 Cal
350 Cal
700 Cal
350 Cal
2,100 Cal Total
2,100 Cal Total

1. Bellisle, F, et al. "Meal frequency and energy balance." *Br J Nutr*, 1997 Apr 77 (Suppl 1): S57-70.
2. Cameron, JD, et al. "Increased meal frequency does not promote greater weight loss in subjects who were prescribed an 8-week eqi-energetic energy-restricted diet." *Br J Nutr*, 2010 Apr 103 (8): 1098-101.
3. Wang, YQ, et al. "Increased eating frequency is associated with lower obesity risk, but higher energy intake in adults: a meta-analysis." *Int J Environ Res Public Health*, 2016 Jun 17; 13 (6): 603.
4. Hutchison, AT and LK Heilbronn. "Metabolic impacts of altering meal frequency and timing—does when we eat matter." *Biochimie*, 2016 May 124: 187-97.
5. Schoenfeld, BJ, et al. "Effects of meal frequency on weight loss and body composition: a meta-analysis." *Nutr Rev*, 2015 Feb 73 (2): 69-82.

7

METABOLISM MYTHS, DEALING WITH A DEFICIT, AND BREAD BREAKS

The oldest recipe for soup included hippopotamus and sparrow meat.

Before we continue on with metabolism myths, I'd like to tell you a story about a modern hunter gather society. The Hadza, who live on the plains of northern Tanzania, survive solely on traditional foraging. There are no supermarkets. No town butcher or bakery. Drive-thrus and fast food are unfathomable. They spend the day either hunting for meat and honey, picking berries and fruit, or digging for tubers. The Hadza construct temporary shelters made of grass and carry all of their possessions on their backs. New camps form around large animal kills, near better hunting grounds, and close to fresh water sources during the dry season.

Sounds like a lot of work. Definitely a lot of movement. How much? The Hadza spend a whopping 135 minutes each day on foraging.[1] Compare that to the *weekly* recommendation of 150 minutes of moderate activity for developed societies.[2] What's even sadder, only about 23% of Americans hit these numbers.[3] It's hard to imagine spending a large part of the day rustling up grub, especially when new apps make it possible to order almost any cuisine with a few taps of the screen.

Navigating camp, walking hunting grounds to stalk prey, and digging for tubers requires Calories. How much, though? Before stumbling across the answer, my best guess ranged between 3,500 and 5,000 Calories per day. Even that seemed like a conservative estimate. What scientists discovered, however, is shocking.

Hadza men burn 2,600 Calories a day, and the women come in around 1,900.[4] These numbers are eerily similar to their Western counterparts. What the what?! You read that correctly. These very active hunter-gathers burn approximately 200-300 more Calories a day (not 2,000-3,000) than your average couch potato.

How is this possible? One hypothesis—total energy expenditure is consistent for a species. Hypothesis is just a swanky word for a specific prediction that needs more investigation. This implies the Calories OUT side of our equation is steady, regardless of where we live and our lifestyles.

All humans roughly burn the same amount of energy. The Hadza use most of their fuel for hunting and gathering. For the rest of us, our energy goes toward BMR. Not buying it? Researchers replicated this phenomenon in other hunger-gather societies and in great apes (by comparing zoo inhabitants to their wild cousins).[5,6]

〜

The Broken Metabolism Myth

You cannot break your metabolism. It is not fragile. You can't throw it against the wall, bash it with a hammer, or hit it with your car. We have mainstream diet media to thank for this nonsense. Charlatans and diet companies capitalize on this misconception. There are pills to "speed it up," coaches convincing clients to "wake it up" in the morning with breakfast, and Sunny Susan selling shaking for "repairing it." You did not break your metabolism. It's doing its job—trying to keep you alive.

Your body's metabolism strives for efficiency.

Put it another way, the body wants to use the least amount of energy to perform the most amount of work. Some say lazy. I say efficient. When food is scarce, metabolism decreases for the sake of survival. There is absolutely no benefit to increase the rate of energy expenditure and risk starvation. For the diet world, this leads us to some uncomfortable truths.

Your body defends against weight loss more than weight gain.

In a modern context where food surrounds us, the struggle is real.

You don't have excess fat because of genetics.

Did mom or dad give you a slower motor? Sure, genetics plays a role. I won't deny it. But so does age. And gender. And skeletal muscle mass. Ultimately, too many Calories are going in and not enough are going out.

Your metabolic rate is variable.

It is just a snapshot in time. Your metabolism will increase or decrease depending on the environment. Adaptation doesn't occur in a single day, but it will occur.

A smaller body burns less energy than a bigger body.

This dovetails with the above statement regarding variability. Your metabolism at the beginning of your weight loss journey will not be the same at the end. It takes more energy to move a bigger body, to feed a bigger body, and to repair a bigger body. Don't believe me. Complete a task with a 20-lb-weighted vest and rate your exertion. Better yet, carry around the number of pounds you've lost on your journey in a backpack for a day. How do you feel?

No particular diet increases metabolism.

Don't spend your hard-earned cash on supplements, super foods, or any product Tricia from high school is hitting you up about on Facebook. Don't buy into this rubbish.

There is no such thing as *starvation* mode.

Humans don't hibernate. We don't horde Calories in the fall to survive the winter in our caves. True starvation is not applicable to weight loss discussions. The swanky term we are looking for here is adaptive thermogenesis—a reduction in metabolism in response to a reduction in Calorie intake. This brings us to our final uncomfortable truth.

Exercise results in a reduction of metabolism, over long periods.

Do you move a lot for your job? Take lots of steps daily? Never skip a training day? Long-term *consistent* TEA links with a plateau in TEE.[7] Your metabolism adapts.

Let's return to our Hadza story. They spend lots of energy during foraging that results in a lower BMR. Compare that to a couch potato who has low energy requirements for movement but a higher metabolism. If we assume the Hadza man burns a similar amount of Calories as an American man, then as a modern society we are not obese because of inactivity—we are obese because we are eating too much.

So you heard, "don't exercise." What I said was "stop eating so much." Exercise is beneficial for all areas of health. Keep moving.

~

How to Survive Hangry

Eating in a caloric deficit sucks. There, I said it. Compared to the joy of shoving fun-filled treats in our piehole, limiting and monitoring our intake is pure drudgery.

If you've followed along my meandering path so far, we should be at the trail marker for "eat fewer Calories to lose weight" near the intersection of "exercise for health benefits."

In theory, this is simple. In real life, this will be very difficult. There will be days when everything is going smoothly and you feel great. Next day, the hunger is almost overwhelming. Fluctuations in scale weight bring a myriad of emotions, and there will be times when it is difficult to visualize the end game. To help you navigate those down times, below is a list of recommendations to avoid the most common pitfalls and keep things as manageable as possible. In corporate lingo, let's set you up for success.

Choose a realistic daily deficit.

Sure, I'd love to burn 2 lbs of fat a week, but living in a 1,000 Calorie daily deficit leaves me with eating air. And ice. And maybe an occasional sprig of lettuce. I don't have the beginning maintenance Calories to support this long-term. What's realistic?

10% daily deficit = acceptable
20% daily deficit = tolerable
30% daily deficit = chew your arm off inadvertently

These are long-term guidelines. I've eaten in a 50% deficit for 2 weeks and didn't kill anyone. Was I happy? NOPE. Did I want to live like that long-term? Double NOPE.

Keep lower Calorie days not less than 50% of higher Calorie days.

When learning to cycle your Calories, I recommend not going too low on the off days. If you follow the Yo-Yo Yak cycle, this is an easy check-and-balance strategy to help calculate your targets.

I'm not a fan of continually cycling the Weekend Whale or Party Pig. These are great for special occasions but can prove problematic long-term.

Just keep swimming.

When eating in a deficit, you will naturally want to move less. Your training numbers can also suffer, if you stay here for too long. What can you do? If you want to train, train. Just be kind to yourself and acknowledge that you are not fueling your body for optimal performance. Otherwise, just walk. Keep your daily step count high.

Program diet breaks and re-feeds.

Notice, I did not say, "cheat meals." These are not excuses to pig out and go crazy. You schedule them in advance with planned targets.

How much and how often? Start small. Eat in a deficit for 3 weeks, then one week at maintenance. Maybe a 2-week-on and 2-week-off plan works best for you. It will take twice as long to lose the scale weight, but it may keep your relationships intact.[8]

Please, please, pretty please (with a cherry on top) remember that it likely took you months to years to store that excess fat. For the sake of your spirit and sanity, give it longer than 6 weeks to lose.

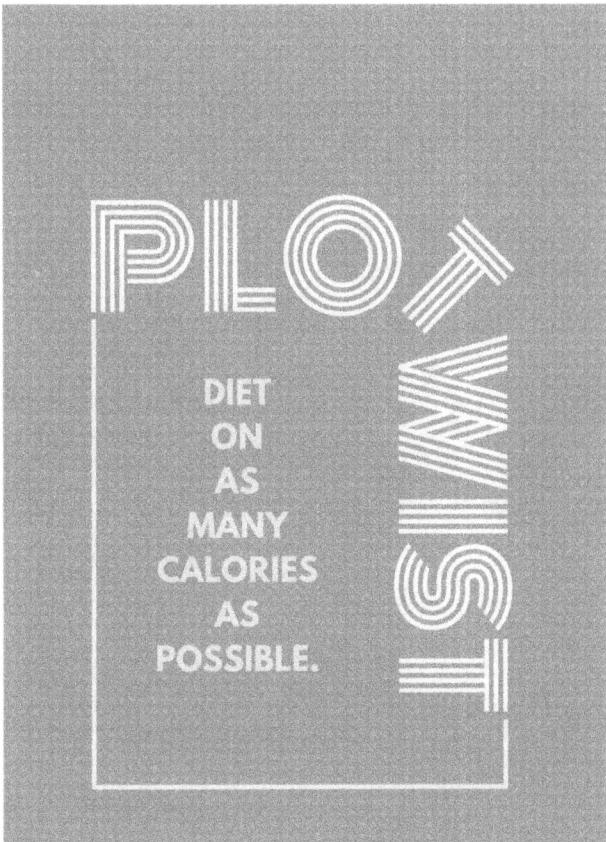

PLOT TWIST

DIET ON AS MANY CALORIES AS POSSIBLE.

1. Pontzer, H, et al. "Energy expenditure and activity among Hadza hunter-gathers." *Am J Hum Biol*, 2015 Sep-Oct 27 (5): 628-37.
2. Recommendations based on the "Physical Activity Guidelines for Americans, 2nd edition." published by the US Department of Health and Human Services.
3. Centers for Disease Control and Prevention, National Center for Health Statistics. Accessed online at https://www.cdc.gov/nchs/fastats/exercise.htm on 02 Oct 2020.
4. Pontzer, H, et al. "Hunter-gather energetic and human obesity." *PLoS One*, 2012 July 7: e40503.
5. Pontzer, H, et al. "Primate energy expenditure and life history." *Proc Natl Acad Sci USA*, 2014 Jan 28; 111 (4): 1433-7.
6. Pontzer, H. "Constrained total energy expenditure and the evolutionary biology of energy balance." *Exerc Sport Sci Rev*, 2015 July 43 (3): 110-6.
7. Pontzer, H, et al. "Constrained total energy expenditure and metabolic adaptation to physical activity in adult humans." *Curr Biol*, 2016 Feb 8; 26 (3): 410-7.

8. Byrne, NM, et al. "Intermittent energy restriction improves weight loss efficiency in obese men: the MATADOR study." *Int J Obes (Lond)*, 2019 Feb 42 (2): 129-138.

8

RAVENOUS, STRESSED-OUT ZOMBIES

In several states, it's illegal to put ice cream in your back pocket.

Our story continues as we return to the 1904 World's Fair in St. Louis. No, there weren't any stressed-out zombies roaming around, but there were a lot of folks clamoring to satisfy their sweet tooth. While the more adventurous tried the new fairy floss, others stuck with a well-known delicacy—ice cream. During the fair, lore has it that one ice cream vendor ran out of tiny serving bowls. In desperation to please his waiting customers, he went to the nearby waffle peddler and convinced him to mold his fare into the funnel-shaped cone similar to what we see today.

Nobody quite knows the exact origin of ice cream. There are stories from Ancient Rome of Nero favoring a combination of snow, fruit, and honey. He often sent messengers into the mountains to gather the frosty ingredients. Another tale reaches us from the Chinese who created a combination of snow, rice, and milk.

The first written recipe of "Icy Cream" dates back to the 1600s. It starts out as expected with a base of cream, sugar, and mace (a spice made from the coverings of nutmeg seeds). For additional flavoring, they added orange flower or ambergris. You may have heard of orange flower, still commonly used as an aromatizer in dessert dishes. Ambergris is a less likely known substance used for its fragrance in candle and perfume making. Found washed up on shore, it is a waxy-gray material created when a sperm whale heaves up a blockage from its small intestines. Personally, I'll take two scoops of Rocky Road and pass on the vanilla-infused whale vomit.

~

Hunger

Ever wonder why it feels more comfortable to stuff yourself with food than to go 20 minutes with a growling tummy? Hunger is the body's defense mechanism against starvation. It's designed as a signaling process to ensure adequate intake of fuel. Hunger manifests from a complex connection between the gut and brain (mainly the hypothalamus). It is purely a response that drives us to find food. Once we are *full*, our brains stop signaling the need to stuff our face.

What about a growling tummy? Where does it fit in with this? Those rumbling noises occur when the stomach is empty. You are hearing peristalsis, a swanky word for involuntary muscle contractions. When the stomach squeezes, the air inside escapes, making the infamous rumbling noises. Like a bagpipe, only just slightly less pleasing to the ears. Contrary to popular belief, empty stomachs don't trigger hunger.

So what does? The answer is our hormones. There are two main hormones that regulate hunger and its opposite—satiety.

Ghrelin is the hunger hormone. Made predominantly in the gut, it signals the brain to eat. Under normal circumstances ghrelin rises before a meal and declines after.

Ever try to fall asleep on an empty stomach? Researchers link levels of ghrelin with our circadian rhythms.[1] Circadian rhythm is just a swanky phrase for our sleep-wake cycle. In other words, the hunger hormone affects our shuteye.

For my menstruating ladies out there, do you ever have crazy cravings associated with certain times in your cycle? Estrogen causes an increase of ghrelin.[2] Super, right?!

Lack of sleep, chronic stress, and long-term Calorie deficits all increase blood levels of our hunger hormone.[3]

Food intake is the most important factor for controlling levels of ghrelin.

~

If hunger drives us to seek food, then satiety tells us to take a break. Leptin is the fullness hormone. Made by fat cells, it signals the brain to stop eating. Leptin lets us know that we have enough energy stores to survive the zombie apocalypse. More fat equals more leptin.

However, some individuals have receptors in the brain that don't respond to increased levels. The swanky term for this is leptin resistance.[4] Think of a broken loop. Your fat says, "I'm big enough," but nothing registers. You never feel full.

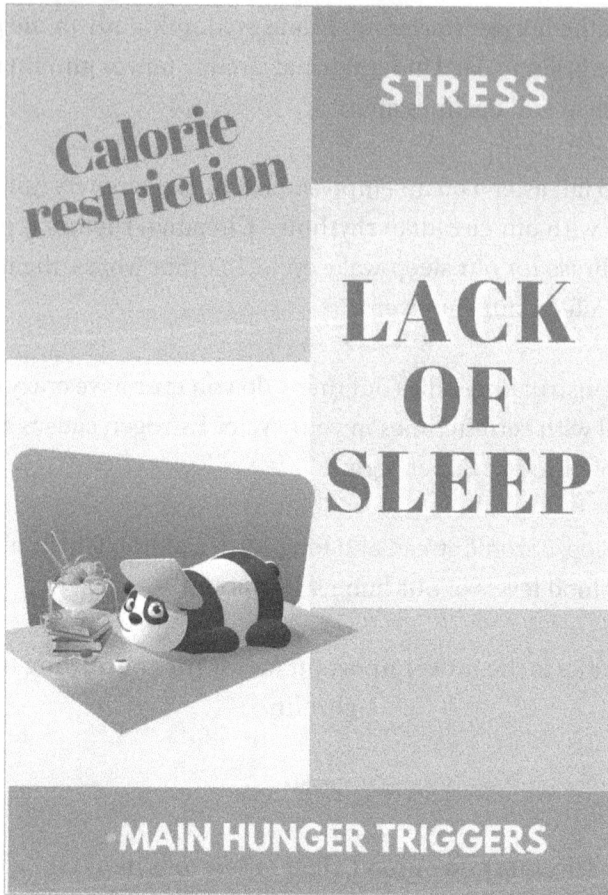

Calorie restriction

STRESS

LACK OF SLEEP

MAIN HUNGER TRIGGERS

Researchers think high levels of inflammation, high levels of fatty acids, and consistently high levels of circulating leptin cause resistance.[5, 6] It's possible the receptors are just plain tired of the constant spamming.

No-Drama Llama:
Drugs or supplements cannot control leptin and ghrelin.

Stop pinning ghrelin as an enemy and leptin as a solution. Reframe your mindset and think of them both as tools the body uses for survival. Instead of searching for a pill, here is a list of the natural ways you can maintain healthy levels of each.

Avoid rapid weight loss.

Scientists measure hormone imbalances a year after crash dieting.[7] It is likely longer but the study had to end sometime. Stop with the extremes. You want to promote the natural rise and fall of ghrelin with mealtimes.

Increase intake of foods that promote feelings of fullness.

Hunger increases when glycogen is low. Eat more fruit. When filled with fat, the stomach empties more slowly.[8] Eat your veggies since fiber slows digestion. Oh, and protein is incredibly satiating.[9, 10]

Manage your stress.

Find your woo-sah. Learn methods of coping that don't include food. This is important for more than just weight loss.

SLEEP!!!

Not enough shut-eye increases cravings, especially for yummy carbs. GO. TO. BED.

Fuel your workouts.

This doesn't mean you can't work out on an empty stomach, but you need to eat enough to fuel your training. Also, prepare for an increase in hunger after a hard session.

Find your personal comfort level for hunger.

Eating in a 10% deficit is manageable. Just grab a snack so you don't snap at your loved ones. At a 20% shortage, hangry is real. Control your urge to get stabby. If you are trying a 30% reduction in Calories, try not to chew off your arm in desperation.

⁓

HAVE you ever made a trip to the grocery store when hungry? What did your cart look like at check out? If it was anything like mine, you likely ended up with the most random assortment of food that wasn't even on your list. I never pick up enough items to put together a meal, but I end up with some cheese, maybe some peanut butter, definitely some chips, and a last-minute candy bar that contains chocolate. My appetite shops for me. This brings us to our next point.

Hunger tells us it's *time to eat*, and our appetite tells us *what to eat*.

Appetite is a sensory reaction that guides our food choices. It is a conditioned response to food affected by sight and smell. Ever start salivating just by looking at something yummy on the TV? That's your appetite. Are you able to leave the last few chips at the bottom of the bag? Food availability affects appetite.[11] If you "sees it, you eats it." Taste also plays a role. If I gave you a plate of plain baked potatoes and one with loaded, twice baked skins, which one do you think you will finish?

Sight, smell, and taste influence appetite.[12]

Your appetite provides the emotional connection to food. It influences your behaviors and leads to changes in your eating habits. Stressed, but not hungry? Appetite steers you to the pantry. Attitudes and perceptions of overall body size also affect your choices.[13] For example, it's not uncommon for young males to want to bulk up. Appetite tells them to keep throwing food down the hatch, even though they feel full. Ever take a stroll down memory lane and suddenly start craving an old favorite snack? The mere recall of food affects our appetites. We see this phenomenon in amnesia patients, too. Unable to remember when they last ate, patients will accept multiple meals, despite the lack of hunger.[14]

Stress, body image, and memories influence appetite.

It is important to distinguish between hunger and appetite. Are you grabbing that sandwich because you need the fuel? Or is your heart telling you to smash that chocolate? Do not overlook your relationship with food. Even though I started with all the science and the maths, this journey is more than just tracking Calories and learning macros. That's why I gave you the 30-day journaling challenge. However, please seek professional guidance if you are experiencing powerful fears or emotions around your eating habits.

~

Stress—Our Cups Runneth Over

I don't know about you, but stress seems to be a constant in my life. Between work, my kiddos, and general adulting, I often fall into bed at night fried from the day. But what is stress? Is it all in our head or is there a physical component to it? Do we need to manage or reduce it? Before I answer these questions, let's cover a little anatomy.

Our first lesson reviews the nervous system.

The nervous system has two branches. We control one—the somatic branch. Getting ready for work, hauling groceries into the house, and cooking for your offspring are examples of voluntary actions of our muscles. We don't have to think about the other branch—the autonomic one. It is responsible for the involuntary actions of our organs. Breathing, circulating blood, or digesting that last bit of breakfast are examples of movements you don't have to pencil in on your thought calendar.

Let's focus in on that automated branch. It controls heart rate, digestion, breathing, salivation, perspiration, pupillary response, urination, and even sexual arousal. Whew. I can't remember why I walked into a room half the time. I'm glad that I don't have to remember to do any of that other stuff.

The automated part of our nervous system has two speeds; go, go, go, and relax. I don't like to use the descriptions "on" and "off" because the system always signals, sometimes just for a slower pace. We also refer to these speeds as "fight-or-flight" and "rest-plus-digest."

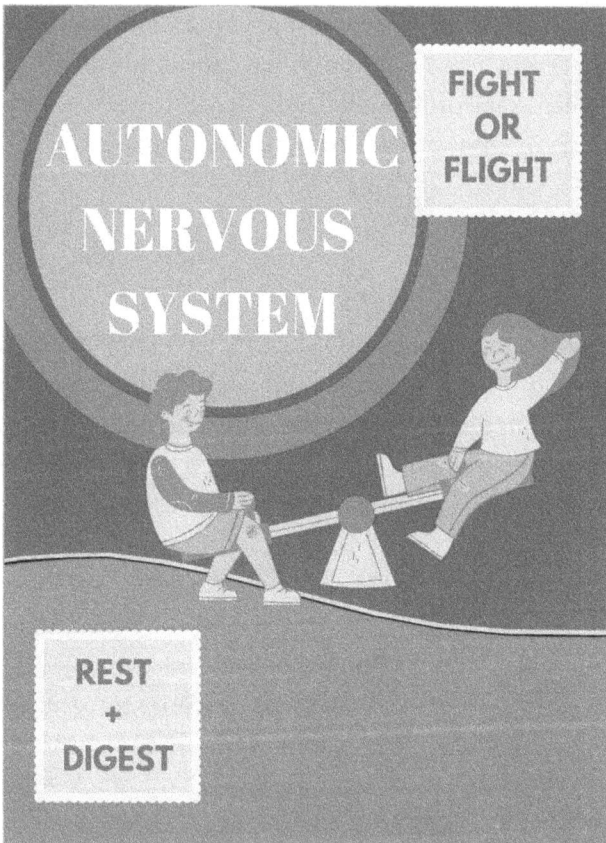

The fight-or-flight response kicks in when we are under stress. It tells us to either stand our ground and fight or get out of harm's way. Our heart and breathing rates increase. The body stops digestion. Our pupils dilate to let in more light. And glucagon breaks down glycogen for extra fuel.

The rest-plus-digest response takes over when there are no threats. It tells us to slow down and chill out. Our heart and breathing rates decrease. The body restarts digestion. Our pupils constrict. We send a signal saying, "stop and use the facilities." Also, now might be a good time to get our hanky-panky on.

Evolutionarily, toggling between "fight-or-flight" and "rest-plus-digest" keeps us alive. Is a lion chasing us? We better turn it up a notch. No predators around? Sweet. Let's eat, or sleep, or practice making babies.

Today, we rarely encounter actual lions. The king of the jungle doesn't roam the streets of downtown waiting outside our workplace. Do you know what *is* on the other side of those doors? Stress—lots and lots of stress. Unfortunately, our automated nervous system can't distinguish between being chased by lions and being cut off in traffic. Nor can it distinguish between a looming work deadline and a stalking grizzly bear. Also, it can't tell the difference between an argument with your significant other and swimming with a great white shark.

The body responds to all stress by activating the fight-or-flight response.

Stress is stress is stress. Don't believe me? Check your pulse after you receive a nasty-gram in your inbox. How steady is your breathing while being honked at in rush hour? I bet you get a spike in your blood glucose levels when dealing with your *strong-willed* toddler. Your body is getting ready to rumble, whether or not there is an actual lion.

What's the big deal? Stress is unavoidable, right? There is nothing inherently wrong with stress. It can light a fire under your booty when you need that extra push. It can keep you alert in dangerous situations like the evening commute. Even lifting weights acts as a stressor on the body, and many enjoy the benefits of the resultant muscle growth. However, a little stress goes a long way. Our bodies need a chance to recover between bouts of crazy.

Stress is beneficial in small doses.

～

What happens when stress is constant? When it never fully dissipates?

This leads us to the second part of our anatomy lesson—stress hormones.

There are three main stress hormones in the body. Adrenaline and noradrenaline trigger the initial phase of the fight-or-flight response and are fast-acting hormones. After the initial "get-up-and-go," the body follows with a release of the hormone cortisol. Think of cortisol release as a maintenance signal, something to sustain the intense energy.

Together, these three hormones serve as the key link between what the brain perceives as a threat and how the body automatically reacts. When their levels return to baseline, our bodies return to default mode—rest-plus-digest.

I want you to picture every movie scene where the hero is lying on the ground, unresponsive. Exposed to sarin gas, the sidekick stabs our hero in the heart with a giant needle that miraculously returns him from the dead. Ever wonder what's in the syringe? It's not an antidote to the poison; it's adrenaline. Adrenaline hits the bloodstream and causes a surge of energy. Heart rate and breathing increase. Pupils widen to let in more light. The body redirects blood toward the larger muscles, and the brain plans an escape route. Alert and focused, our hero lives to save the day.

Contrast this fast-paced action, with the slower response of cortisol. Cortisol release occurs in minutes instead of seconds. Once the hormone is in circulation, it maintains fluid balance and blood pressure, decreases libido, and halts digestion. That is all fine and dandy in the short-term because we don't want to waste precious energy to make a baby or take a dump.

With movie magic, the hero contains the threat. Theater-goers relax in their seats. We get a happily ever after or a promise of a sequel. In reality, too many never get that chance to wind down. Their cups of stress runneth over.

There are consequences to chronically high levels of stress and cortisol production. Over time, cortisol suppresses the immune system, which makes it more difficult to fight off infections.[15] It also elevates blood pressure, increases blood glucose levels, and decreases libido. That's no fun for mama, either. Cortisol works with your circadian rhythm and sleep patterns. Higher levels at bedtime make it more difficult to fall and stay asleep.[16, 17] Finally, scientists link chronically high levels of cortisol with obesity.[18, 19, 20]

Depressing, right?! Proper management of stress is beyond this book. If you need professional guidance, many resources are available. Please find them. Use them. Incorporate their practices.

In the meantime, let's live by the adage, "knowledge is power." Stress influences weight. The link is undeniable. I implore you to address your stress before you ever track a macro.

~

Counting Sheep

Too many consider sleep a luxury. We live a fast-paced existence and try to wring every ounce of life out of the time given. There are only 24 hours in a day, and we only live once. YOLO, right? Cleaning up your sleeping habits is the most important step in your weight loss journey. You read that right. SLEEP. Sure, our body requires a Calorie deficit to lose mass, but you will not sustain long-term weight loss until you fix your sleep.

Fixing your sleep is the most important step on your weight loss journey.

It's a bold stance for a diet book, but here's why:

The Unicorn Diet **is a lifestyle change.**

AND

Health is more important than scale weight.

Sure, I want you to reach your weight loss goals. But changing your lifestyle for the better is more important than a quick reduction in scale weight. So without further ado, here are the top ten reasons for a proper night's rest.

1. It is vital to our immune system.[21, 22]
Sleep helps restore our immune cells, and it decreases susceptibility to disease.

2. It is important for learning.
Studying for an exam? Our brains organize memories during shut-eye. Learn a new trick? The new motor pathway gets mapped at night.

3. It leads to improved cognition.[23, 24]

Cognition is just a swanky word for getting smarter. It includes our concentration and decision-making skills. Who doesn't want to be better at board games and adulting?

4. It is responsible for tissue recovery.

Our body and mind recover during sleep. See also: we don't make muscles in the gym. Training sends the signal, but they grow during recovery.

5. It is necessary for tissue repair.

During sleep, the body releases hormones that encourage tissue repair. Wounds heal faster, and the body rebuilds damaged muscles.

6. It contributes to the balance of sex hormones.[25, 26]

In both men and women, sleep helps balance levels of testosterone. Testosterone signals the body to make new things instead of breaking them down.

7. It improves athletic performance.[27]

Fatigue from lack of sleep decreases power, speed, and accuracy. Nobody likes a weak teammate.

8. It affects blood glucose levels.[28, 29]

Not getting enough sleep? Our cells stop responding to insulin. Remember, we need insulin to direct our energy storage.

9. IT CHANGES THE WAY YOUR BODY INTERPRETS HUNGER SIGNALS.[30, 31]

This is a double whammy. Too little sleep causes an increase in hunger. Hello again, ghrelin. It also causes a decrease in leptin, the fullness hormone. Recall, long-term sleep deprivation is likely one mechanism for developing leptin resistance.

10. IT IS STONGLY LINKED WITH WEIGHT GAIN.[32, 33]
Not getting enough sleep is one of the strongest risk factors for obesity. It probably feels like I'm yelling at you with my bolded list and shout-y capitals. Well, I am. GET TO BED.

How much sleep do we need? That depends on genetics and age, but the current recommendation for people 18 to 64 years old is 7 to 9 hours and for folks 65 and older 7 to 8 hours.[34]

Aim for 8 hours of quality sleep per night.

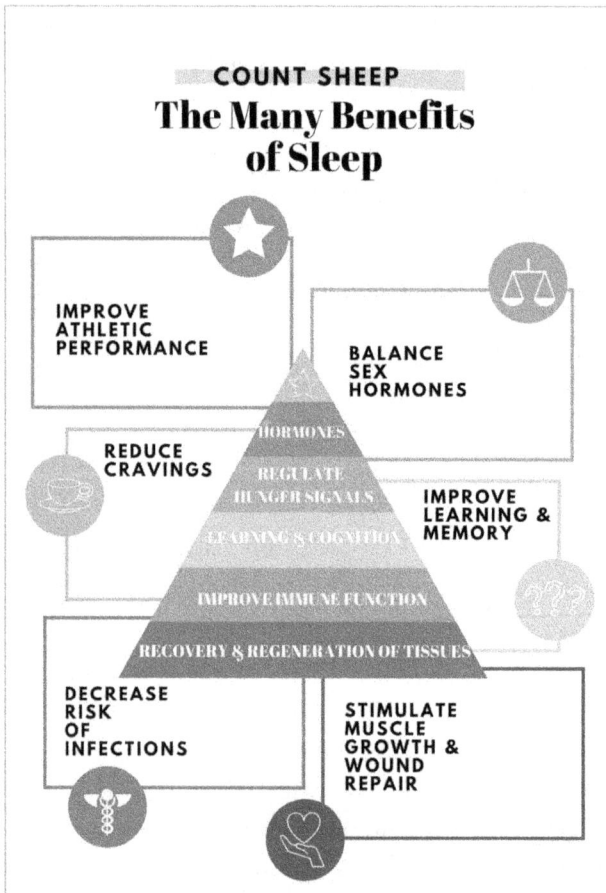

COUNT SHEEP
The Many Benefits of Sleep

IMPROVE ATHLETIC PERFORMANCE

BALANCE SEX HORMONES

REDUCE CRAVINGS

IMPROVE LEARNING & MEMORY

HORMONES

REGULATE HUNGER SIGNALS

LEARNING & COGNITION

IMPROVE IMMUNE FUNCTION

RECOVERY & REGENERATION OF TISSUES

DECREASE RISK OF INFECTIONS

STIMULATE MUSCLE GROWTH & WOUND REPAIR

Now that we've covered the importance of sleep, I will leave you with some tips and tricks to improve both the quantity and quality of your snooze.

1) Establish a bedtime routine and a morning routine.
This includes going to bed and getting up at roughly the same time every day. At night, eliminate excess lighting and electronics one hour before slumber. Do you find it too difficult to break the screen habit? Wear blue light blocking glasses and use minimal ambient lighting before you snooze.

2) Eliminate caffeine after your mid-day point.
Sure, tolerance and genetics play a significant role in how your body metabolizes caffeine, but the vast majority of us would benefit from just cutting off the bean juice after the lunch hour.

3) Develop the practice of 2-minute-box breathing.
There are plenty of tutorials online showing proper techniques. This can be a game changer for managing stress and relaxing the body for bedtime.

4) Use this opportunity to complete your journaling.
Let go of your worries and find your happy moments.

5) Reduce or eliminate alcohol consumption at bedtime.
Sure, alcohol may help you crash or fall asleep initially, but it interferes with brain waves and disrupts sleep patterns, which can leave you feeling exhausted in the morning.

In a world full of zombies, be a unicorn.

---

1. Klok, MD, et al. "The role of leptin and ghrelin in the regulation of food intake and body weight in humans: a review." *Obes Rev*, 2007 Jan 8 (1): 21-34.
2. Müller, TD, et al. "Ghrelin." *Mol Metab*, 2015 Mar 21; 4 (6): 437-60.

3. Chaput, JP, et al. "Obesity: a disease or a biological adaptation? An update." *Obes Rev*, 2012 Aug 13 (8): 681-91.

4. Considine, RV, et al. "Serum immunoreactive-leptin concentrations in normal-weight and obese humans." *N Engl J Med*, 1996 Feb 1; 334 (5): 292-5.

5. Park, HK and RS Ahima. "Physiology of leptin: energy homeostasis, neuroendocrine function and metabolism." *Metab*, 2015 Jan 64 (1): 24-34.

6. Jung, CH and MS Kim. "Molecular mechanisms of central leptin resistance in obesity." *Arch Pharm Res*, 2013 Feb 36 (2): 201-7.

7. Sumithran, P, et al. "Long-term persistence of hormonal adaptations to weight loss." *N Engl J Med*, 2011 Oct 27; 365 (17): 1597-604.

8. Parra, D, et al. "A diet rich in long chain Omega-3 fatty acids modulates satiety in overweight and obese volunteers during weight loss." *Appet*, 2008 Nov 51 (3): 676-680.

9. Westerterp-Plantenga, MS, et al. "Dietary protein—its role in satiety, energentics, weight loss and health." *Br J Nutr*, 2012 Aug 108 (Suppl 2): S105-12.

10. Chambers, L, et al. "Optimising foods for satiety." *Tren in Food Sci & Tech*, 2015 Feb 41 (2): 149-160.

11. Wansink, B, et al. "Ice cream illusions bowls, spoons, and self-served portion sizes." *Am J Prev Med*, 2006 Sep 31 (3): 240-3.

12. Rogers, PJ and JM Brunstrom. "Appetite and energy balancing." *Physiol Behav*, 2016 Oct 1; 164 (Pt B): 465-71.

13. Oliveria, N, et al. "Association of body image (dis)satisfaction and perception with food consumption according to the NOVA classification: Pró-Saúde study." *Appet*, 2020 Jan 1; (144): 1044-64.

14. Higgs, S, et al. "Sensory-specific satiety is intact in amnesics who eat multiple meals." *Psychol Sci*, 2008 Jul 19 (7): 623-8.

15. Buford, TW and DS Willoughby. "Impact of DHEA(S) and cortisol on immune function in again: a brief review." *Appl Physiol Nutr Metab*, 2008 Jun 33 (3): 429-33.

16. Pistollato, F, et al. "Associations between sleep, cortisol regulation, and diet: possible implications for the risk of Alzheimer disease." *Adv Nutr*, 2016 Jul 15; 7 (4): 679-89.

17. Powell, Daniel JH, et al. "Unstimulated cortisol secretory activity in everyday life and its relationship with fatigue and chronic fatigue syndrome: a systematic review and subset meta-analysis." *Psychoneuroendo*, 2013 Nov 38 (11): 2405-22.

18. Spencer, SJ and A Tilbrook. "The glucocorticoid contribution to obesity." *Stress*, 2011 May 14 (3): 233-46.

19. Vicennati, V, et al. "Stress-related development of obesity and cortisol in women." *Obesity*, 2009 Sep 17 (9): 1678-83.

20. Lee, MJ, et al. "Deconstructing the roles of glucocorticoids in adipose tissue biology and the development of central obesity." *Biochem Biophys Acta*, 2014 Mar 1842 (3): 473-81.

21. Cohen S, et al. "Sleep habits and susceptibility to the common cold." *Arch Intern Med*, 2009 Jan 12; 169 (1): 62-67.

22. Prather, AA et al. "Behaviorally assessed sleep and susceptibility to the common cold." *Sleep*, 2015 Sep 1; 38 (9): 1353-9.

23. Ellenbogen, JM. "Cognitive benefits of sleep and their loss due to sleep deprivation." *Neurology*, 2005 Apr 12; 64 (7): E25-7.

24. Könen, T, et al. "Cognitive benefits of last night's sleep: daily variations in children's sleep behavior are related to working memory fluctuations." *J Child Psychol Psychiatry*, 2015 Feb 56 (2): 171-82.

25. Burschtin, O and J Wang. "Testosterone deficiency and sleep apnea." *Sleep Med Clin*, 2016 Dec 11 (4): 525-529.

26. Lo, EM, et al. "Alternatives to testosterone therapy: a review." *Sex Med Rev*, 2018 Jan 6 (1): 106-113.

27. Vitale, KC, et al. "Sleep hygiene for optimizing recovery in athletes: review and recommendations." *Int J Sports Med*, 2019 Aug 40 (8): 535-543.

28. van Leeuwen, WM, et al. "Prolonged sleep restriction affects glucose metabolism in healthy young men." *Int J Endocrinol*, 2010 Apr 19: 108641.

29. Rao, MN, et al. "Subchronic sleep restriction causes tissue-specific insulin resistance." *J CLin Endocrionol Metab.* 2015 Apr 100 (4): 1664-71.

30. Taheri, S, et al. "Short sleep duration is associated with reduced leptin, elevated ghrelin, and increased body mass index." *PLoS Med*, 2004 Dec 1 (3): e62.

31. Markwald, RR, et al. "Impact of insufficient sleep on total daily energy expenditure, food intake, and weight gain." *Proc Natl Acad Sci USA*, 2013 Apr 1; 110 (14): 5695-700.

32. Patel, SR and FB Hu. "Short sleep duration and weight gain: a systematic review." *Obesity*, 2008 Mar 16 (3): 643-53.

33. Ogilvie, RP and SR Patel. "The epidemiology of sleep and obesity." *Sleep Health*, 2017 Oct 3 (5): 383-388.

34. Hirshkowitz, M, et al. "National sleep foundation's sleep time duration recommendations: methodology and results summary." *Sleep Health*, 2015 Mar 1 (1): 40-43.

9

CORPORATE LINGO MAKES MY EARS BLEED

Arachibutyrophobia is the fear of peanut butter sticking to your mouth.

On average, Americans consume 6 lbs of peanuts per person per year. Of those 6 lbs, we devour a whooping 50% in the form of spreadable butter. Smeared with jelly on white bread for a childhood staple. Swirls of gooey goodness in candy and frozen treats. Eating it straight out of the container lollipop-style. And for the more sophisticated among us, used as a base in savory dishes. It's hard to imagine a food culture without the presence of the tasty legume.

Historians trace the origins of the plant back to South America, some 3,500 years ago. Like any fabulous food, their existence flourished with trade routes. Let's follow the peanut's path around the globe. First, Europeans "discovered" them in Brazil and brought them home to Spain. Then they quickly spread to Asia and Africa. Finally, they travelled back across the Atlantic Ocean to North America. Peanuts became prominent in the states after the American Civil War when

Union soldiers brought them home. Their popularity as a snack item soared with PT Barnum's traveling circus.

What about peanut butter? In my childhood history lessons, my teachers erroneously credited Dr. George Washington Carver with its invention. South American Inca Indians are the earliest society believed to have ground peanuts into a spreadable paste. In the United States, our good friend Dr. Kellogg created a version as a protein source for the elderly with poor teeth. Peanut butter was introduced alongside fairy floss and ice cream cones at the 1904 World's Fair in St. Louis. But what about Dr. Carver? It pleased me to learn that he is responsible for something even greater.

Born as a slave in Missouri in 1864, George Washington Carver was a somewhat sickly child and unable to work in the fields. He took to wandering about the woods near his home. Through observation, keen intellect, and natural curiosity, he quickly became known as the resident "plant doctor." Dr. Carver completed his formal education at Iowa State University, where he was both the first black student and the first black faculty member. Later in his career, Booker T. Washington recruited him to head the Agricultural department at Tuskegee Institute in Alabama.

In his lab at Tuskegee, Dr. Carver and his graduate students conducted research on ways to separate fats, oils, sugars, gums, and resins that resulted in the discovery of over 300 uses for peanuts! They successfully teased out recipes for caramels, chili sauce, and coffee. His group found uses for peanuts in cosmetics for shampoo, shaving cream, and lotions. We can trace its incorporation into household items, glues, and plastics to his lab. In 1916, Dr. Carver wrote a bulletin titled, "How to Grow the Peanut and 105 Ways of Preparing It for Human Consumption." And when the boll weevil destroyed Alabama's cotton fields, that titillating thriller provided the "how-to" guide for converting peanuts to a cash crop. While we should not credit Dr. George Washington Carver for inventing peanut butter, we must give him kudos for saving the entire economy of The South.

~

Don't Work in a Silo—
The Overlap of Aesthetics, Performance, and Health

Why are you on this journey? Do you want to look better in a bikini? Maybe you need to survive running a 5K for your kid's school fundraiser. What about reducing the amount of medication you take every morning? How about all three?

Improvements in aesthetics, physical performance, and health are not always independent outcomes. Losing excess fat, putting on some muscle, and finding a hobby that increases daily movement will often benefit all three areas.

However, there are extremes to this triad. The football player, who shows up to work on any given Sunday, risks long-term brain damage from concussions. As an elite athlete, he is at the pinnacle of performance, but there is a toll to his physical well-being. What about your friend with the 8-pack? Sure, she looks great with her shirt off, but her questionable eating habits are wrecking hormone levels.

What's more important to you? Is it health, aesthetics, or performance? It is possible to improve all three, but watch out for the extremes.

Here are two questions that you should ask yourself periodically.

1) What is my primary goal?

AND

2) Can I live with the sacrifices?

Let's use my midlife crisis to illustrate how these questions shape our actions along the way. Somewhere in my mid-30s, I had the spark of motivation to shed the extra baby weight that I had been carrying around from two pregnancies. I say "baby weight" but in reality my youngest was 6 years old.

For almost a decade, I let my exercise routine slide. My eating habits changed for the worse while trying to wrangle two young children and finish professional school. That's me, the stress eater. So I did what many do in this situation. I joined a new gym.

But it wasn't just any ole commercial gym. Nope. I joined a mixed martial arts studio. If I was going to spend a good chunk of time away from my family and pay someone to make me sore all over, I wanted to learn a new skill set.

It started off as you might imagine. I regularly attended evening kick-boxing classes taught by pro fighters. They were grueling, but they hooked me on the thrill of learning new movement patterns. Fast-forward 6 months. I looked around and realized that I lost the new kid status. I no longer needed to ask the instructors to repeat the punch combination. Other regulars started seeking me out during warm-ups to partner in class.

The weight did not melt off as quickly as it did in my early 20s. However, my pants fit better, and I could play with my daughters without my body protesting the next day. Let's return to our two questions.

My primary goal was to lose weight and learn a new skill set.

AND

The sacrifice of time and money was worth the result.

Another 6 months passed and the instructors invited me to join the advanced class. Instead of using pads, I graduated to kicking and punching my classmates. My focus shifted from throwing punches for weight loss to mastery of common combos, proper blocking, and creative counter attacks.

Fast-forward a few more months and my instructors asked if I have any interest in live sparring. Live sparring?! We kick and punch each other for realsies? I was crazy enough to try. Like a rock rolling downhill, I accepted my first amateur kickboxing bout a mere 12 months after my fitness lightening strike.

Sure, I was nervous about stepping in the ring. In front of actual humans. To trade blows with a stranger. There was one teeny, tiny detail that made me want to run in the other direction.

My competition was for a catch weight of 150 lbs. Unfortunately, I walked around at 165 lbs. Eek. I had to make it through the end-of-year holidays and somehow figure out how to lose those 15 lbs of baby weight in 5 months. Until that point, I had only lost a half a pound a week, at most.

But how? All of my prior weight loss had been purely organic, with a little luck, and a dash of common sense. So I did what any person would do in my situation. I asked Dr. Google. You can probably guess what I found. Turd nugget after turd nugget after turd nugget.

Sure, I'd love to just drink a shake to "wake up my metabolism." Let me spend my hard-earned cash on cling wrap to melt away the belly fat. And who doesn't want to pee expensive supplements?

Fed up trying to find the answers on my own, I ended up hiring a coach. Our brief relationship lasted only 3 months. During that time, we found my maintenance Calories. He taught me how to use a kitchen scale, how to log my food, and how to take body measurements. My coach was my accountability partner. Those weekly check-ins kept me on the path to success. We parted ways, and I continued my journey alone, using the tools he imparted. Returning to our two questions,

My primary goal was to not become a YouTube sensation by KO.

AND

The sacrifice of time and money was worth the result.

Two fights and 1 year later, I accepted my third match in the 135 lb weight class. You read that right. A full 30 lbs down from the weight where my body felt comfortable.

I lost the pounds and for the first time in my life, and I had abs. I'm not talking about a 6-pack or the defined hint of obliques. Nope. I had a beautiful 8-pack washboard. You could have cleaned the grass stains out of your son's white baseball pants on my tummy-tum-tum. My arms, shoulders, and back could have served as an inspiration for sculptors. In short, I was cut, ripped or shredded, as the kids are calling it these days.

After my win, that magnificent body lasted all of 2 weeks. Why? Why go to all that trouble then blow it? Well, what had happened was... I like tasty things. Give me a cold, hard cider on a hot day. Pile on some pulled pork and extra helpings of potato salad for a dinner date. Oh, I always have room for dessert, especially pie. I'm not talking about a slice. Anything under ¼ of the pan will not cut it.

To my dismay, my personal energy expenditure does not allow for super-dense, high-calorie goodies every day, even when I'm training like a fiend. Back to our two questions.

My primary goal was to bring home the win.

AND

The sacrifice of my sanity and the strain on my personal relationships were not worth it.

Every so often, it's important to re-examine your goals. I had to take a step back from training and focus on my health and my family. It's okay to change your direction. Take a moment to realign your priorities, and start a new goal if needed. You are not a failure for chasing happiness.

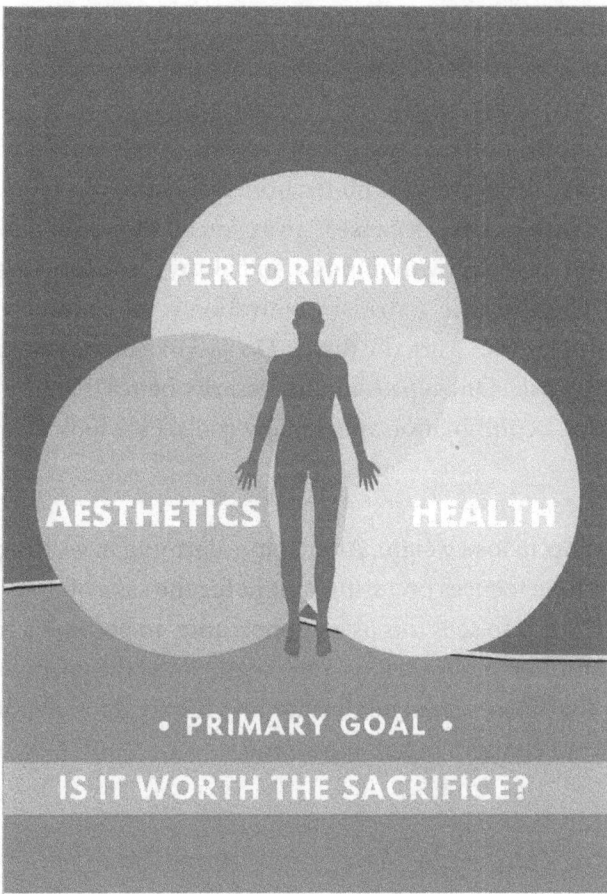

PERFORMANCE

AESTHETICS HEALTH

• PRIMARY GOAL •

IS IT WORTH THE SACRIFICE?

～

Stick to Core Competencies—Habits Trump Motivation

Over the years, friends have asked me many times, "how do you motivate yourself to go to the gym?" Another one I commonly encounter is "how do you have the willpower to stick to your diet?"

Motivation is a tricky subject and also very personal. What might work for me may not strike a fire under someone else. To be clear, I'm not referring to fleeting desires. You may run across an Insta-famous model and think "hey, I wish my <insert body part here> looked like that." That quick tickle of your senses rarely spurs action. But what does? What is motivation? And how can we use it to reach our goals?

We divide motivation into two categories—Intrinsic and Extrinsic. Internal rewards drive intrinsic motivation. For example, you may help a neighbor with a chore because it gives you all the warm and fuzzy feels. Do you have a growth mindset and always look for ways to improve? Also, intrinsic. Extrinsic motivation is the counterpart. Here, external rewards are the driver. Do you like money or praise? Both are extrinsic. One type is not necessarily better than the other. In fact, a combination spurs many goals. Let's look at an example.

> Julie wants to lose weight. After some alarming news from her doctor, Julie focuses on losing weight for the sake of health. She also sees this as an opportunity to become a role model for her children. Plus, Julie really loves the positive praise that comes from her friends and family upon making significant changes in her appearance.

～

There are five types of intrinsic motivation. I have listed them below with examples of each.

Competence or Learning Motivation:
Crave the process rather than the reward at the end

Even though I started kickboxing to lose weight, I quickly felt motivated to learn a new skill. I thrived on the challenge of mastering new combos. I enjoyed working with new partners and speaking with my instructors on their philosophy of combat. After a few months into my new hobby, this became my primary motivation.

Attitude Motivation:
The desire to change the way you (or others) think and feel

I love this motivation. When used positively, it results in a large change in perception of self and can carry through to all areas of daily living. How do you approach weight loss? Are you Sara, mom to 3 kids, or are you an athlete, training and honing your body? How do you think your training session at the gym will go in each of these cases? I bet Sara, the athlete, beats, Sara, the mom, any day of the week.

Achievement Motivation:
Value the process rather than the result

Think of every movie montage. We see our hero transforming her body or learning her craft in a series of knitted scenes. Cue the motivational music. It doesn't really matter what happens at the end. Maybe our hero wins the boxing match. Or she loses the championship game. The viewer knows all is well in the universe because our hero transformed in the process and can now weather any outcome.

Creative Motivation:
The need to express yourself

There is an artist inside all of us. For some, that internal creative is bursting with expression. Writing, painting, or singing for sheer joy is motivation for many. They may never create a hit single on the radio or sell their paintings to support their family, but that's not the point. Creating for the sake of expression alone is their jam.

Physiological Motivation:
Our body and mind have certain physical needs

We need food. And a roof over our heads. And safety. And health. Be watchful for negative drivers in this category. It's natural and all too easy to let fear and anxiety creep in here.

$$\sim$$

There are four types of extrinsic motivation. I have listed them below with examples of each.

Incentive Motivation:
The reward is the reward

Incentive motivation is the counterpart to achievement motivation. The outcome, as opposed to the process, is the driver. In my case, winning my last kickboxing match was more important than the achievement of stepping in the ring. Another example is gaining new skills for your job. Instead of being proud of the personal accomplishment, the associated pay raise is the primary reason you took all those accounting courses or stayed late and worked on an extra project.

Power Motivation:
The wish to establish control over self or others

There are plenty of examples in both history and fiction of individuals motivated by power over others. Think dictators and villains. These are the obvious extremes. What about power of choice? There is a certain allure to being the owner of your actions. Instead of allowing a diet plan to *tell you* what you can and can't eat, reframe your mindset such that you are *choosing* to eat more fruits and veggies. It's switching from "my diet doesn't allow for break room cookies," to "I'm choosing to eat healthier today."

Fear Motivation:
The fear as fuel for action

Fear can be a driver for motivation, but it can also lead to unhealthy behaviors. Obsessive thoughts, trouble sleeping, and inability to perform activities of daily living are on one end of the fear spectrum. On the other end, we can use fear as a positive stressor, to improve or outsmart our future self. For example, the fear of what you might look like in a bikini may drive you to make positive changes now. As long as that fear is not all consuming, we can use it as a motivator for changing present behaviors.

Affliction and Social Motivation:
The desire to belong

Humans have an innate desire to bond and connect with others. We are quick to form groups and are more likely to exhibit behaviors that bolster or maintain our status in the tribe. I have mom friends, industry friends, workout friends, gardening friends, and childhood friends. Each group has its own dynamic and social constructs. My gym friends hold a special piece of my heart. We have a mutual obligation to each other to show up and give our undivided attention every week, regardless of how tired we may be, or how stressed our day has been, or how much we would rather just put on our fluffy pajamas and drink our evening meal on the couch.

∽

What's your motivation? What are your drivers? Have you ever said them out loud? Ever written them down? Unleashed them into the universe?

Homework time: Go back to that journal and make some notes about motivation and your personal drivers. Keep in mind that you may have a couple. For example, your reason for participating in a new sport may be a combination of achievement motivation (intrinsic) and social motivation (extrinsic). Be sure to explore your motivation for changing your diet, and your motivators for starting a new exercise program or hobby. The drivers for each may be different, even though the end goal of a healthy body may be the same.

∽

Many moons ago, as a young, baby-faced teenager, I made some extra spending money watching a handful of neighborhood kids. One of my very first jobs was for a family of four. My initial gig was to watch their two young daughters for an evening, allowing the parents a much-needed date night. As instructed, I arrived a few minutes early that first night to acquaint myself with their bedtime routine, go over an orientation of the house, and review the list of important emergency numbers.

Mom showed no concern regarding my skills to keep her darlings alive. She did, however, have doubts about my capability for enforcing the nightly teeth-brushing regimen. Apparently, there was a history of rebellion during this chore. So much so, that the parents went out to the bookstore and purchased a very large color coffee-table book named something along the lines of "The Book of British Smiles."[1] It only took a few pages to convince the girls to polish their pearly whites.

Questionable parenting aside, why do you brush your teeth every day? Is it the fear of incrimination every 6 months when visiting the dentist? Or maybe a beautiful smile motivates you. How far does motivation take you first thing in the morning before your first cup of caffeine bean juice? How high is your motivation to scrub those pearly whites right before bed when you just want to keel over from exhaustion?

Habits trump motivation on days of the week that end in–y. Motivation will light the fire, but establishing habits will lead to behavior change. There are 5 keys to success when forming new habits.

1) Schedule it!

To create a new habit, we must make space in our life to accommodate it. Sounds like a straightforward decision. However, this is the most overlooked step.

Want to run a marathon? Outstanding. How many days a week are you training? Four. That's great. But what days this week? What times? Wait, it's already Friday, and you didn't run once! It's going to be hard to hit your goal of 4 runs with only 3 days left in the week.

WRITE. IT. DOWN. Make a date with yourself. Repeat the next week and then the next.

2) Take small bites.

Setting lofty goals from day one is another barrier to success. Do not misinterpret my words as "aim low." Consider a realistic timeframe to accomplish your feat.

Jumping back to our marathon example, what if you are not a runner? Start by making the habit of running 1 mile a few times a week. Repeat. Increase your mileage slowly or follow a training plan. Entering a 26.2-mile race 2 months after starting running is just crazy talk. Take a few months to establish the habit before you spend your money on an entrance fee. Corporate lingo makes my ears bleed, but it's important to set yourself up for success. Or, as my grandma would say, "don't bite off more than you can chew."

3) Incorporate the habit into your identity.

This is another important step for reframing your mindset. "I'm on a diet," sounds restrictive. It comes across as the habit itself, controlling and limiting your actions. Instead, identify as a healthy eater. "I'm choosing to eat this healthy meal to fuel my workout." Your new persona will assist your decision making on the days you find it hard to continue.

4) Put accountability into action.

Accountability is just a swanky term for accepting responsibility for yo' self. Newer habits are not a part of our routine. They may not yet be a part of our identity.

Accountability leads to a healthy growth mindset. Are you meeting your goals? Have you taken ownership of the change in your life? How are you measuring success and failures?

Holding yourself accountable for establishing habits is one way to meet your goals. It's important to encourage yourself along the journey and to be your own personal cheerleader. Don't criticize.

My rule of thumb: if you wouldn't say it to your child or your pet, don't say it to yourself.

Next form a safety net or accountability team. This could be an individual, such as a family member or friend. Or it could be a group on Facebook or at the gym. If finances allow, hiring a coach or qualified trainer is a fantastic way to incorporate an impartial observer and is often money well spent.

5) Consider your timeframe.

Forming a habit in 21 days is a myth.

It can take anywhere from 2 to 8 months to form a habit.[2]

For some, going through the motions above is not enough. They may still require a crucial moment—an "aha" so big that it leads them to making a very difficult lifelong change.

There is no magic number of days, nor minimum amount of time. I'm not telling you this to be a Negative Nellie. I'm aiming for quite the opposite, actually.

Be kind to yourself. Acknowledge your failures. Don't use them as an excuse to quit. Dust yourself off and get back up on that horse.

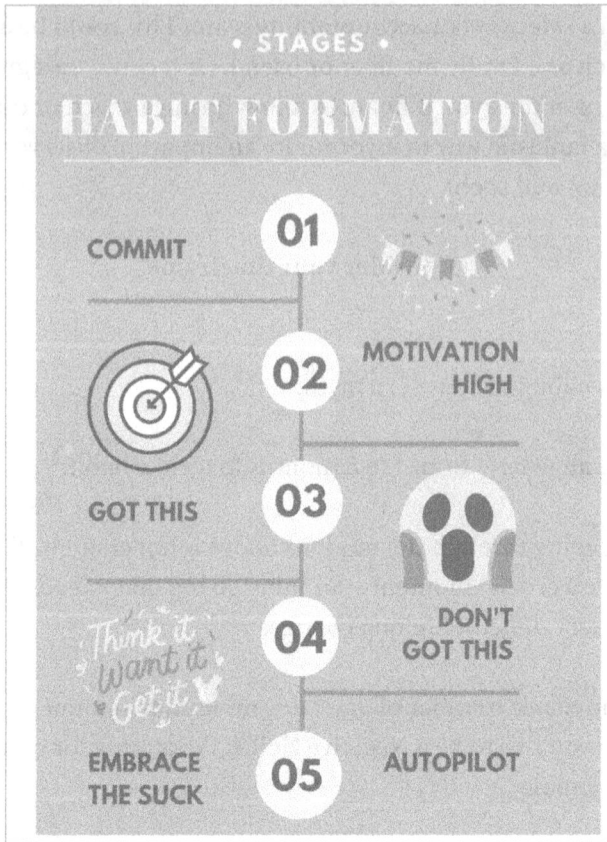

STAGES

HABIT FORMATION

COMMIT — 01

02 — MOTIVATION HIGH

GOT THIS — 03

04 — DON'T GOT THIS

EMBRACE THE SUCK — 05 — AUTOPILOT

Think it want it Get it

Paradigm Shift—A New Blueprint

It's ironic and by design that I'm placing the blueprint for *The Unicorn Diet* at the very end of the book. Hopefully, you've taken the direct route to get here. Your eyes may have glossed over while reading protein structure and function. I may have lost you on the different ways to log ingredients into an app. Maybe you completely bypassed my section intros. They were my attempt to spice things up a little, but I realize some of you just wanted to get to the meat and potatoes.

Did you look at the table of contents and click the link to get here? Just read the intro and skipped to the climax? Maybe you tried the macro section but couldn't grit it out. Go back. Read what you missed. Consider a fresh perspective on *what you think you know*. Otherwise, you will miss the most important theme of this story.

This is not a calorie-counting diet;
it is a rallying cry to change your lifestyle.

But, but you said, "All diets work because of a Calorie deficit."

Yeppers.

"Didn't you spend all that time teaching us how to log, track, and measure?"

You betcha.

"AGGGGH. You made me do the maths, find targets, and adjust percentages."

<Raises Hand> #guiltyascharged

These are all crucial, along with sleep, managing stress, and increasing movement. Looking at your relationship with food may be even more important.

Knowledge is power. Learning the science of weight loss is essential. You also need an ounce of common sense. And the wisdom to understand that you can't possibly tackle all of my recommendations at once.

Where does that leave us? The starting point.

Pick 1-3 items off the homework list, and start today.

Notice I didn't say 5, or 7, or ALL OF THEM.

Now write them down. These are your new goals, and they deserve to be free in the universe.

Next, brainstorm the behavior changes necessary to meet those goals. Write these changes down underneath each goal.

Now, find a calendar with enough space for each day to make notes and document compliance. Did you meet your goal? A simple check mark will suffice. What were your struggles or barriers to success? Add those, too.

Let's reframe your mindset from making excuses to acknowledging obstacles and brainstorming solutions.

Put a star on your calendar 3 weeks into the future. I can feel you rolling your eyes because I just told you in the last section that the 21-day rule for habits was a myth. Still, we have to pick a timeframe to assess our progress. Two weeks is too short and a month may be just enough time to fall off the wagon.

How did you do? Look at each goal individually. Did you establish daily habits that made it easy to meet your target? How many days were you able to put a check mark on the calendar? Was it 19 out of 21? Or closer to 12? Is this a change that you can easily continue in your lifestyle or did it feel like a grind every single day?

It's decision-tree time.

**If you successfully met all your goals,
pick 1-3 new ones to add to the list.**

OR

**If you met 2 goals but not the third, add 1-2 new goals and KEEP
the original one that is not quite a habit.**

OR

**If you did not consistently meet any of the goals, do not add new
ones.**

This last decision point is tricky and requires a very hard look. Maybe
you picked 3 very difficult goals to start. This is very common when
everyone is riding the initial wave of motivation. My suggestion is to
keep one of your original goals and just work on it singularly. Too
hard to stomach? Pick one or two easy goals that require little
behavior change to go along with the big one. This should satisfy
your inner desire to check off boxes on the calendar each day. Let's
look at an example.

Meet Kayla.
Kayla wants to start strong with *The Unicorn Diet*.
Go, Kayla.
She picks three goals and marks her calendar 21 days into the
future.
Kayla begins the eating habit journal.
She tracks her current Calorie intake.
Kayla weighs herself daily.
At 21 days, Kayla feels overwhelmed.
She had 18 check marks for scale weight, 15 for her eating
habits journal, and 7 for Calorie tracking.
Kayla continues to weigh herself.

She continues her journal.
But she stops tracking her Calorie intake.
Kayla recognizes some steps she missed. She needs to learn
how to read a nutrition label and use a food scale first.
Be like Kayla.

Remember, *The Unicorn Diet* is a lifestyle change. Be kind to yourself
and start with manageable changes. Revise. Add slowly.

I will say it again. Your body didn't change overnight, so stop with the
6-week nonsense. Or even the 90-day crap. Don't spend your hard
earned cash on quick fixes, "superfoods," or a MULTI-LEVEL
MARKETING scheme. Let's all jump off this Yo-Yo diet wagon and
live our best life.

---

1. I do not know the actual title of the book. It contained many photographs of
    gnarly smiles. I do remember wondering why they only included individuals
    from one country.
2. Lally P, et al. "How are habits formed: modeling habit formation in the real
    world." *Eur J Soc Psychol*, 2010 Oct 40: 998-1009.

10

THE HOMEWORK LIST

Eggplants are fruit, considered by some to be a berry.

Note: These are in the order they appear in the book. You don't have to follow them as steps. As always, you do you, boo.

1) Make a list of your favorite protein sources. Extra credit for foods that contain essential amino acids.

2) Make a list of excellent sources of Omega-3s.

3) Reduce consumption of Omega-6s.

4) Make a list of 10 high-fiber fruits and veggies, ones that you will eat!

5) Discuss vitamin deficiencies with your primary care provider.

6) Increase your water intake.

7) Complete the Venn Diagram challenge. Is it a protein, carb, or fat?

8) Learn how to read a nutrition label.

9) Buy a food scale and use it.

10) Practice weighing dry ingredients, wet ingredients, and solids.

11) Start meal prepping and determining the Calories of large batches of food.

12) Make a list of your favorite sauces. Which ones are low in Calories? Medium? High?

13) Buy a bathroom scale and start tracking your weight.

14) Buy a soft tape measure and learn how to take body measurements.

15) Start taking progress photos.

16) Define your relationship with food. WRITE IT DOWN.

17) Start a 30-day eating habit journal.

18) Schedule movement.

19) Track your steps. Increase your goal by 2,000 every week until you reach 10,000 steps daily.

20) Track your menstrual cycle, not just shark week.

21) Journal your worries twice a week.

22) Start daily acknowledgements of 5 positive things.

23) Choose a weekly deficit target.

24) Determine maintenance Calories.

25) Calculate weekly Calories (Maintenance - Deficit).

26) Pick an animal strategy and calculate daily Calorie targets from weekly pot.

27) Calculate and track protein goals.

28) Calculate and track fat goals.

29) Calculate and track carb goals.

30) Wear a weighted vest equal to your current fat loss. Repeat every so often.

31) Establish a morning routine.

32) Establish a bedtime routine.

33) Eliminate caffeine after lunch.

34) Learn 2-minute box or belly breathing. Practice at bedtime.

35) Reduce alcohol consumption before sleep.

36) Explore your motivators for change. Write them down.

37) Define your primary goal for weight loss? Is it health, aesthetics, or performance?

38) Take a step back and determine if you can live with these changes.

39) Schedule new habits at the beginning of the week.

40) Establish a realistic game plan for your new habits.

41) Incorporate your new habits into your identity. Write them down. SAY THEM OUT LOUD.

42) Hold yourself accountable. Need help? Enlist a friend, coach, or partner.

43) JUST
44) BREATHE
45) AND
46) BE
47) KIND
48) TO
49) YOURSELF.
50) THE END.

AFTERWORD

Thank you for reading my book. I hope you found something useful among all of the terrible jokes, weird food facts, and goofy slang.

Best of luck on your mythical quest, dear Unicorn.

You can reach out, sign up for my newsletter, or poke around in my sandbox at https://www.mklorber.com.

Love it? Hate it? Find my words, just meh? Please consider leaving a review. I'd love to hear your thoughts and perspectives. Good, bad, or indifferent, I appreciate *all* forms of feedback!

ABOUT THE AUTHOR

Melissa Kay Lorber is the leading authority on nothing. Nada. Zip, zero, zilch.

Melissa is an optometrist by day and an introvert by night. A mid-life crisis led to an undefeated (3-0) career as an amateur kickboxer. Her four kids are convinced she was put on this earth to embarrass them. She has just the right amount of dogs (at three), not enough cats (only one), and is still trying to convince her other half that they *need* goats. And chickens. MK lives in the armpit of the Midwest (St. Louis, Missouri) with her partner-in-crime and their crazy circus.

www.ingramcontent.com/pod-product-compliance
Lightning Source LLC
Chambersburg PA
CBHW060336030426
42336CB00011B/1363